T0261802

Using Hypnosis With Children

More Advance Praise for
Using Hypnosis with Children

"This book is an amazing resource and learning tool for anyone working hypnotically with children—both seasoned clinicians and those just developing their skills in hypnosis. It blends Lyons' wisdom, creativity, knowledge, and skill gleaned from her years as a gifted psychotherapist to create an interventional framework to use when working with children. The result is a toolbox full of clever strategies, useful techniques, and magical metaphors to stimulate our own creativity when working hypnotically to help children help themselves."

—**Linda Thomson, PhD, APRN, ABMH, ABHN**,
Past President, American Society of Clinical Hypnosis

"This book is quite special. It contains practical suggestions for both the novice and the experienced clinician who is already using hypnosis. Sensible approaches for children of all developmental levels, as well as their parents, are described. With this book, Lynn Lyons has made a valuable contribution to the field of pediatric hypnosis."

—**Jeffrey E. Lazarus, MD, FAAP**, former Associate Clinical Professor, Case Western University School of Medicine; Pediatrician specializing in medical hypnosis in Menlo Park, California

A Norton Professional Book

Using Hypnosis With Children

Creating and Delivering
Effective Interventions

Lynn Lyons

Foreword by Michael D. Yapko

W.W. Norton & Company
New York • London

Copyright © 2015 by Lynn Lyons

For information about permission to reproduce selections from this book,
write to Permissions, W. W. Norton & Company, Inc.,
500 Fifth Avenue, New York, NY 10110

For information about special discounts for bulk purchases, please contact
W. W. Norton Special Sales at specialsales@wwnorton.com or 800-233-4830

Manufacturing by Edwards Brothers Malloy
Production manager: Christine Critelli

Library of Congress Cataloging-in-Publication Data

Lyons, Lynn.
Using hypnosis with children : creating and delivering effective interventions /
Lynn Lyons ; foreword by Michael D. Yapko. — First edition.
      pages cm
Includes bibliographical references and index.
ISBN 978-0-393-70899-8 (hardcover : alk. paper)
1. Hypnotism—Therapeutic use. 2. Child psychotherapy. I. Title.
RJ505.H86L96 2015
615.8'512083—dc23

                                                            2015022950

W. W. Norton & Company, Inc.
500 Fifth Avenue, New York, N.Y. 10110
www.wwnorton.com

W. W. Norton & Company Ltd.
Castle House, 75/76 Wells Street, London W1T 3QT

1 2 3 4 5 6 7 8 9 0

To my parents,
Ed and Cathleen Gerwig,
who listen to my stories.

Contents

Contents

Foreword

Michael D. Yapko

*K*ids are struggling, and so are their parents, many of whom are learning the hard way that no matter how much bubble wrap they want to protectively cushion their child with, it's not enough. Besides, the bubble wrap itself becomes part of the problem when an overprotected child is unprepared for the rude awakening he or she will have when discovering the world isn't going to protect him or her the way Mom or Dad did. Kids need support, information, and practical tools if they are to not only survive but thrive in today's complicated world.

While young people of every generation have inevitably had to face the ongoing challenges of life, in recent years these challenges have taken on new, unprecedented forms. These include school shootings, bullying and cyberbullying, virtual rather than real friendships, kids kidnapped right off the street and sexually abused or even murdered, families fragmenting, a fragile and unstable economy that leaves too many kids in poverty or close to it, and on and on. Young people face an intensity and complexity while just trying to grow up that not enough people truly understand to be of much help to them.

The mental health statistics reveal the consequences of these relentless stressors on our kids: millions of children are on psychiatric medications, especially antidepressants and antianxiety drugs that are themselves problematic because of their side effects and largely unknown effects on children's neurological, physical, and social development; excessive caseloads in middle school, high school, and college counseling centers that struggle with a level of demand that far outweighs their collective supply; and kids just suffering in silence, ignored by adults who are much too busy to notice them until they act out, act up, or simply give up acting altogether and withdraw into despair.

With this superb book, psychotherapist and pediatric specialist Lynn Lyons offers genuine help to all those young people—and their families—so desperately in need. Lyons possesses an infectious optimism, a persuasive "you can do it!" attitude that I'm confident therapists can absorb and share with their young clients. It's a powerful attitude that can set the foundation for absorbing the meaningful growth Lyons's practical methods can catalyze.

On the surface, this is a book about integrating clinical hypnosis into one's treatment of children and adolescents. On just that level alone, this book succeeds in a very big way, for Lyons teaches us with clarity and skill the artistry of constructing and delivering therapeutic hypnosis sessions with kids for many of the most common problems they face. She reviews salient clinical literature and shares it in a clear and compelling way. She carefully emphasizes the absolute necessity of adapting one's hypnosis sessions to the uniqueness of each child, including his or her developmental considerations, interests, experiences, hopes, important relationships, and more. Beyond that, Lyons provides plenty of clear and instructive examples of what to actually say before, during, and after hypnosis sessions, sharing her knowledge and artistry most generously. Her ability not just to do hypnosis but also to be hypnotic is nothing short of inspiring, for the delivery style and specific language she uses and teaches so skillfully serve as a true role model of what good therapy utilizing hypnosis can look like and ultimately achieve. Lyons provides current and convincing examples of why it's so important for therapists to pay attention to attention, a core component of both hypnosis and effective living.

Beneath the surface, this book is about much more than pediatric hypnosis. It's about empowering young people to begin to develop some vision and the skills to bring those visions to fruition. Lyons is consistent in her key messages embedded throughout the book: kids are capable of more; kids have innate resources to be tapped into and directed toward meaningful goals; kids are much more than their symptoms or their diagnosis; and kids are naturally oriented toward growth, especially evident when therapists and others provide the means and support for facilitating that growth. So much of what Lyons describes in this book is ways to use language and relationship to get these key messages across to young people so desperate to hear and absorb them.

Lyons is a realist. She makes it crystal clear how critically important it is to work not only with kids, but also with their families. In that sense, this book is as much about the skills of effective parenting as it is about conducting hypnosis sessions with young people. Lyons provides many compelling examples of the kinds of suggestions that support parents but also challenge them to be deliberate in soothing and inspiring their children. This is a wonderful gift that will undoubtedly keep on giving over the family's lifetime.

Pediatric hypnosis is a specialty in its own right and Lynn Lyons is one of its leading advocates. Interest in pediatric hypnosis has been steadily increasing in recent years as more and more practitioners recognize the need for specialized approaches to treating children as well as the value of hypnosis as an empowering treatment approach. Empowering children to use their imaginations and creatively solve problems, develop life-enhancing skills, and think and act more effectively are critically important benefits of employing hypnosis. Lyons provides a solid consideration of practical issues associated with applying hypnosis from how and when to introduce it to how to structure sessions for maximum benefit. Lyons has written an excellent how-to book that fulfills its promise to make therapists better at doing therapy when they learn and apply the hypnotic approaches she describes.

Lynn Lyons has made an enormously valuable contribution to a too-small body of literature on the subject of pediatric hypnosis. Her expertise is apparent on every page and we are fortunate she shares it so generously. I hope and expect this book will be widely read and thoughtfully considered, and as a result will prompt more child and adolescent psychotherapists to pursue training in clinical hypnosis. Kids urgently need the help that these gentle and empowering methods can provide.

Through this book, Lynn Lyons has given us the gift of a compelling vision of how thoughtful words can heal. Perhaps best of all, she has given every therapist who works with kids a chance to share in that vision.

Acknowledgments

At its core, this is a book about connecting to what we need most, on the inside and the outside. I am acutely aware of the connections that sustained me as I worked on this project and that mean so much to me as I move through my personal and professional life.

First and foremost, I am thankful for my husband, Crawford, and my boys, Brackett and Zed. Every day we laugh. We tell stories and jokes, come up with terrible puns, and know that humor and silliness and guffawing are the stuff of our family's best moments together. There are finite hours in a day, and my boys gave me many as I worked on this book. They were understanding, patient, independent, and loving from start to finish.

My parents, Cathleen and Ed Gerwig, have been married for 52 years and continue to show their family what connection looks like. My love and gratitude for all they have taught and given me is hard to express in words. I think they know. My siblings, Nancy, Ed, and Robin and their incredible children are truly gifts in my life.

As is clear throughout this book, Michael Yapko's contributions to the psychotherapy and hypnosis field are remarkable, and his generosity to me has been constant. He helped shape my career and this book. I hope he knows the place he holds in my heart as a mentor, cheerleader, and friend.

My collaboration and friendship with Reid Wilson has made me a better therapist and a happier human being. He raises my game with his creativity, openness, humor, and brilliance.

Jeffrey Zeig has been inspiring and supportive, and I am deeply grateful. The Rigmor House gang has become, over the past decade, a group of cherished friends. Being together is one of the highlights of my year. Christine Cook remains the friend who defines the word *friend*. Jay Essif got the ball rolling and 22 years later I still feel lucky.

For many years, I have started my days with the support and humor of my early morning workout and biking pals and our amazing trainer, Brian. Sweat, laughter, and sunrises make any project easier to tackle.

Thanks to my dentist, Charles Albee, and my physician friends, Paul Urbanek and Michael Lynch, for their expertise. Julie Bassi offered her input and support, and as a school psychologist is modeling and teaching connection to children every day. Mary Buckley Raine and Bill and Judy Egan have a special place in our family's heart for their gentle, creative, and hypnotic gifts. To have your children taught by such virtuosos is valuable beyond measure. All parents should have such amazing role models.

Deborah Malmud at times appeared clairvoyant in her ability to take what I said and make it better. Thank you to Deborah and her team at Norton for all their help and commitment to this book.

And finally, thank you to all of the children and parents who give me the honor of sharing in their stories and listening to mine.

CHAPTER *1*

Why Use Hypnosis With Children?

*I*f you work with children in one of the many helping professions, then you help families find solutions. As a therapist or guidance counselor, you help anxious, depressed, or confused kids navigate all sorts of family, social, and school-related challenges. If you're in the medical field, children and parents look to you to diagnose and treat their illnesses and injuries, alleviate their suffering, and help them recover and feel better.

Sometimes these struggling children and their parents come to you in a heightened state, worried or unsure or angry, spinning with thoughts and feelings and even conflict as they work to understand what's happening and how to fix it. And sometimes they arrive exhausted and skeptical. They're still searching, but the pace has slowed. The frenetic spin of "what's wrong?" has moved toward the deflated shrug of "why bother?" In either case, the goal is to help discover, create, and then use the resources they need to get back on track. There are many different ways to achieve this. The book you are holding focuses on one of them: hypnosis.

The goal of this book is to enhance your effectiveness with children by elevating your use of hypnosis as a treatment tool. Of course, you can no sooner become skilled at hypnosis by only reading a book than you can call yourself a builder after only studying blueprints. This book is for those who have some training and exposure to hypnosis and want to improve their skills and their confidence. My job is to sharpen your own clinical practice by walking you through a step-by-step process that shows you how to create and deliver tailored interventions from start to finish. Ultimately, I hope you'll be inspired to incorporate hypnotic techniques and language, formally and informally, and make them an integral part of your interactions with families.

Imagine how you'll enhance your work with children when you:

- Increase your ability to identify the pattern of problems presented
- Use hypnotic language and interventions to engage and connect with children and amplify their resources from the very first contact
- Creatively offer new or alternative frames that will move the child toward the desired outcome
- Gain the confidence to use hypnosis with children more frequently and with more versatility
- Teach children a skill they can use to manage their current struggle and then use more broadly thereafter to prevent and handle issues as they move through life

Now you might be saying to yourself, "Well, isn't that what all solution-focused therapy does? Hypnosis doesn't own the rights to helping children access strengths and make positive changes." And I couldn't agree more, because hypnosis, in my opinion and in the opinion of many past and contemporary experts, is not a treatment or therapy in and of itself, but a tool that can help children and adults discover the best parts of themselves, and then use those resources to cope and thrive.

So what is hypnosis with children? Why use hypnosis with children? What makes it different—or even more effective—than any other tool? In this first chapter, before we move into the specifics of creating meaningful hypnotic interventions, let's address these questions. I want you to be excited about the value of hypnosis in a child's contemporary world, and to appreciate how this versatile tool creates wonderful opportunities for the children and teens you see.

WHAT IS HYPNOSIS WITH CHILDREN?

Defining hypnosis with children is a tricky proposition, as it is with adults. Decades of research have examined facets of the hypnotic encounter in order to more clearly understand what makes hypnosis effective (Kirsch, 2000, 2005a; Barber, 2000; Lynn & Sherman, 2000; Lynn, Fassler, & Knox, 2005).

Admittedly, I've given a lot of thought to the question, "What constitutes hypnosis with children?" Certainly, if I've written a book on the use of hypnosis with children, I must believe there are properties and qualities that make it distinct from other approaches. On the other hand, my experience of being with children in both a clinical setting and as a mother in a world surrounded by kids reminds me constantly that children, simply because they are tasked with growing and learning and deciphering, are consistently in the process of focusing, absorbing, and organizing their internal and external experiences. As Yapko wrote, "Hypnosis can be found in other places than hypnosis" (2012, p. 516), and this is certainly nowhere truer than in the realm of treating children.

Perhaps clinical hypnosis with children is best broadly understood as the deliberate utilization of this naturally occurring trance-like state—this developmental mandate to use absorption, fantasy, and imaginative rehearsal—as a way to help a child move forward by discovering his own resources and capabilities, and then more specifically to learn new skills and apply them. I therefore define my use of hypnosis with children in the following way:

> *I am using hypnosis with a child when I am able to absorb and join a child in an imaginative experience that allows us to alter sensations, change perceptions, shift a perspective, and discover a solution together. The experience itself, the posthypnotic suggestions, and the practicing that follows allow the child to then apply these new skills and perspectives to future situations.*

When children tell stories, draw pictures, build with Legos, or pretend to be a cat, they are engaging in what we might refer to as a trancelike state, absorbed in their imaginations and unrestricted by the laws of the "real world." We expect and accept this aspect of how children learn and explore. Sugarman and Wester aptly stated, "It is not so much that children are 'good at hypnosis'; more aptly they live, full time, in the trance of intense psychophysiological development" (2013, p. 7).

THE VALUE OF TAKING ACTION

This is not an easy time to be a child. Although I'm sure many previous generations have legitimately made the same claim, the increasing rates of anxiety, depression, attention problems, and obesity, and the increased use of psychiatric medications in children and adolescents (Mojtabai & Olfson, 2010; Thomas, Conrad, Casler, & Goodman, 2006; Schubart, Camacho, & Leslie, 2014) are uniquely modern problems and perhaps indicative of the stress our culture manufactures and the approaches to managing such stress.

My philosophy as a therapist—which will reappear again and

again as you read this book—is to consistently simplify, clarify, and move my clients to action. Anxious, concerned families tend to be rigid and catastrophic in their thinking. Therefore, from the very first contact, I want to shift them out of crisis and reactivity mode and into problem solving (Wilson & Lyons, 2013). If a child has been to other appointments or therapists, must endure tests or medical procedures, or is having trouble functioning at home and school, there's a good chance that everyone is feeling on edge. Introducing and then incorporating the experience of hypnosis can help create flexibility and establish a framework for the solution-focused work to come.

To answer the general question, "Why use hypnosis?" I describe below three overarching advantages to using hypnosis as a tool to help children. You'll recognize these general principles woven throughout the upcoming chapters, reappearing as we move through the process of creating more specific interventions.

Hypnosis Can (Quickly) Change or Establish the Emotional Tone of the Therapy

When 11-year-old Kyle arrived for his first visit, he had already been out of school for 8 months. He had seen other therapists, his pediatrician, and a specialist, all trying to convince him that his stomachaches were from anxiety, or "all in his head," as he reported. His arms were crossed tightly across his chest as he blinked back angry tears. "I don't know for sure what's happening with your stomach yet, but I can tell you're stressed," I said. "Can I show you something that will help you feel better right now, loosen up your muscles, and then we can figure out what to do next?"

Hypnosis offers an experience that for many children and parents is different from the pace they've been keeping as they deal with a chronic problem or new crisis. Kids and parents find that slowing down, focusing their attention in a different way, and taking a break from the current struggle serves as an important respite and alternative to strong emotional reactions. In the span of a few minutes, Kyle had the experience of being able to shift from anger and defensiveness to feeling calmer and at ease. He now had a refuge and a taste of a new skill. Did our first brief process together stop his stomachaches right away? No, but it allowed us to move in a positive direction, and for Kyle and me to have a different quality of interaction. By the end of the session, Kyle and I were playing one of his favorite songs on my computer, and he was showing me his dance moves; he arrived happily for the second session, reporting that he was back in school. During subsequent sessions, we used hypnosis to help shift his anxious thinking and his perceptions of his stomach pain. And we also did some dancing.

Hypnosis provides the opportunity for play and humor, allowing a family to see the work of therapy and change as interesting—even fun—and the problems they face as manageable. Anxiety in particular loves to be taken seriously, and withers in the face of humor and levity (Lyons, 2013). Hypnosis can provide a context for play and silliness, as you help a child elicit his playful imagination to sing to the worry under his bed. Or how about some clever wordplay with an eighth grader who vomits before baseball practice that talks about all the different types of throwing (out, in, up, around) and how some types are more helpful than others. As Jay Haley (2015) said, "A therapist must be serious about the grim situation of his clientele while being free to change the framework of the situation in the spirit of play."

Hypnosis Is Experiential

Lizbeth met me at the pediatrician's office, and we sat together in the examining room. We had met once before at my office a few days earlier. "I need a meningitis vaccine to attend col-

lege and I leave in two weeks," Lizbeth told me at that first meeting. "But every time I go into the doctor's office, I end up running out like a 4-year-old when they call my name." Lizbeth and I did a hypnosis session in my office, and recorded it, and she listened to it a few times before her vaccine appointment. As we waited for the nurse, I asked Lizbeth to close her eyes, go inside, and remember our session. "What message is most meaningful at this moment?" I asked her. "I am 18 and ready to go off to college. I have a mature part of me that has learned how to handle the childlike fears that pop up in all of us. My mature part can stay here and get the job done, even if the scared part wants to get up and run." Just as we rehearsed, she sat with her eyes closed, and allowed the nurse to give her the shot.

This book is, first and foremost, a book of action. This might surprise most people, based on the common vision of hypnosis as still, quiet, or passive. Many equate hypnosis with relaxation, which isn't wrong, but, in the context of helping children (and adults, as well), too limited. I view hypnosis as a tool that helps someone get from here to there. Hypnosis is a bridge from stuck to solutions. When you use hypnosis effectively, something happens. Something shifts. When I use hypnosis with children, there may be moments of stillness, but in the larger frame of helping families, it's all about inducing movement—sometimes literally, as Kyle would attest.

Introducing behavioral activation as a component of treatment improves outcomes and participation (Lejuez, Hopko, & Hopko, 2001), and hypnosis is an experience that promotes the value of action in a few significant ways. First, the hypnotic encounter itself is active and engaging. Children are not passive recipients, but participants, using their imaginations, their bodies, their senses, and their voices to create the session with the therapist. Second, hypnosis can and should be used as a way to seed therapeutic homework assignments (Haley, 1973; Zeig, 1990; Yapko, 2012) or prepare for actual events. In fact, the hypnosis you do with children is the rehearsal for a later experience out in the world. Children may rehearse how to talk to themselves before a test or how to handle their anxious ruminations about getting lost. They may learn how to dissociate from their bodies during a medical procedure, or how to connect to their bodies while learning something in occupational therapy.

Offering an engaging experience early in treatment also helps to shift expectations and worries about what therapy will be like, enhancing that important emotional shift I described above. Children often expect therapy to be boring and anticipate being subjected to intrusive or uncomfortable questions and examination. Parents' expectations vary from hopeful to desperate to resigned. Many are weary of telling their story to another professional and expect therapy to be all talk. Often they have been through an assessment in which they offer information, but then must wait until a future meeting for treatment to occur. Using hypnosis in the initial session shows a family that we are going to do something and immediately creates positive momentum toward action and improvement.

Hypnosis Promotes Mastery

Kimberly stood at the end of the diving board, three feet above the water. She bounced a little, but her body was careful and stiff. Her toes curled over the end of the board as her father treaded water below her. They'd already had many conversations about how it all worked: how deep she would go when she hit the water, the need to blow air out of her nose to keep water from going up her nose, the short distance she knew she could swim to the side of the pool. Now both were silent. Kimberly's eyes were fixed on the water, in a squint that made her forehead wrinkle. Bounce. Bounce. Finally, Kimberly's father gently spoke: "The first jump is the toughest. Just get the first time over with." Without looking up, Kimberly said, "It's not the first time, Daddy. I've already jumped eight times in my mind."

As I mentioned previously, one of the most tenacious misconceptions about hypnosis is that the person doing the hypnosis is controlling the person receiving it. This is based on media depictions and stage hypnotists, swinging a pendulum and convincing seemingly reasonable people to do silly things. The opposite tenet is what makes hypnosis with children so powerful: hypnosis is in fact a vehicle that promotes mastery and creates self-control. Using hypnosis, a child can mentally rehearse, physiologically change, cognitively shift, and emotionally regulate. A child who discovers the capacity to go inside and pull out what he needs moves into our uncertain world saying, "I don't know exactly what will happen next, but I can handle it."

Hypnosis creates problem solvers who can cope more independently with a variety of challenges, both physical and emotional. A child who must endure repeated blood draws—and has no choice in the matter—can master the ability to make his arm numb, or to feel the needle and respond to it in a different way. A child who becomes overwhelmed by the chaos and noise level on the typical school bus ride can learn how to shift her focus away from the background noise and absorb herself in a positive experience of her choosing. A child who must adapt to her parents' divorce can, in the context of a session with an attentive therapist, recall the loving supports that have helped her in the past, and visualize how she will use them again in her present situation. These abilities taught to a child set the stage for future successes throughout life. Jerome Kagan writes of the power of mastery in his book *The Human Spark*: "The belief that one has some control over daily experiences is one of the best predictors of life satisfaction among adults in most societies" (2013, p. 89).

Emotionally and cognitively, we can show children how to view themselves and their challenges through a different framework. Hypnosis prompts kids to search for alternative paths and different (more positive) outcomes, and then connects the new framework to real events. We can use hypnosis to say to a family, "There might be another solution, another way to move forward." And stuck families need this alternative lens of possibility. Research on anxious children and their parents shows that such families benefit from improving problem-solving skills and increasing autonomy in the family system (Ginsburg, 2009). Martin Seligman (1995, 2011) has created successful programs that bring optimism into schools, giving parents and teachers the tools that shift children toward meaningful, pleasant, and engaging experiences.

Hypnosis promotes mastery concretely by helping a child fall asleep in her own bed or regain her focus during an important exam. But once a child experiences a confidence boost from handling a specific circumstance, we can then help her to generalize this ability. How did you find a solution? What did you do to take control? What do you know about yourself now that you didn't know before? And where will you use that knowledge again in the future? Anxious children dismiss or forget past victories, and therefore benefit from connecting back to their successes as they move into new experiences (Wilson & Lyons, 2013). Depressed children, overwhelmed by their sadness, can reconnect to times when they felt happier and optimistic, and bring those memories into the present (Kohen & Murray, 2006).

Perhaps most importantly, children and teens living in this quickly changing world develop mastery through a process of better thinking. As Yapko wrote, "The greatest preventative tool you can teach a child is the ability to think critically" (2009, p. 180). I hope as you read this book you will discover that each specific problem you address with hypnosis creates a versatile template for teaching the broader skills that children need to thrive and succeed.

The value of teaching these skills to children and their potential for prevention with children was made more poignant for me recently when I met Ingrid.

Ingrid came to see me just shy of her 60th birthday. Quietly, as she looked down at her shoes, she described a lifelong history of anxiety and depression. She spent her childhood—and most of her time since—nervous and afraid. There were hospitalizations and medications, and many therapists along the way. Relationships suffered, and her husband and grown children were frustrated and worn out. She didn't have a job, but wanted one. She sought me out for hypnosis for a specific and fairly new phobia because she had read that hypnosis might work for such things. She was tired, she said, and she wanted some freedom.

We did a hypnosis session together during that first meeting. The messages I offered her through my suggestions and metaphors were nothing new to me. Anxiety and phobias are my specialty. But when Ingrid opened her eyes, she made and held eye contact with me. "I've never looked at my fears that way before," she said. "I even feel hopeful. If only you had taught me that when I was 8."

WHO SHOULD DO HYPNOSIS—AND WHO SHOULDN'T?

The decision to use hypnosis with a child should be made with the same clinical judgment used for any other treatment decision. Hypnosis and being hypnotic can be used in so many different settings and circumstances; therefore, its integration into your work with children must be based on your scope of practice and experience in these settings. If you are not trained or licensed to treat depression in children, then you are not qualified to use hypnosis in the treatment of depression in children. While you may be trained in the treatment of chronic pain, you may not be capable of diagnosing the source of a physical symptom or advocating the use of hypnosis as a way to eliminate a symptom without proper evaluations.

I urge you to be fully informed and collaborative when dealing with a child's physical issues. Hypnosis is a terrific tool to help children with asthma, headaches, surgical preparation, irritable bowel syndrome, and many other physical issues (e.g., Drake & Ginsburg, 2012a; Kuttner, 2012; Baumann, 2002) as I discuss in Chapter 8. But assuming that a child's symptoms are emotional or behavioral, without a proper medical evaluation, is irresponsible. Olness and Libbey (1987) found that 20% of children referred for hypnotherapy for behavioral health issues actually had an organic basis for their symptoms.

I also think there is a danger in overselling hypnosis. Wanting to enthusiastically promote its value is a tempting reaction against those who dismiss it as New Agey or entertainment, but a balanced view that supports hypnosis as a highly effective therapeutic tool and an adjunct to other treatment adds to its credibility. Those of us who experience the value of hypnosis want to prove its effectiveness and versatility to others, but we must avoid advocating for its use when another treatment may be a better choice (Kohen & Olness, 2011).

For example, a few years ago a mother was hopeful that I could teach her daughter to use hypnosis as a way to manage a dental procedure without Novocaine because the girl was afraid of the injection. Both were excited about the idea, having seen a show demonstrating hypnosis during surgery. However, the dentist and I agreed that this was not the circumstance to try out a newly acquired skill. We worked instead on using hypnosis skills to manage her anxiety about the injection of Novocaine, a better option for her and the dentist. In my experience, when hypnosis is viewed as a part of the overall treatment approach, rather than the exclusive treatment, its value and effectiveness are greatly appreciated by all involved and increase the odds of successful outcomes.

Clinicians who specialize in hypnosis often provide information on their websites. It's an opportunity to demystify the experience by outlining the process and answering common questions. If you are going to receive referrals and wish others to recognize you as someone who does hypnosis as the core of your practice, then providing such information can be efficient and helpful.

Some clinicians recommend the use of reading material (like brochures) combined with the signing of a specific consent form giving you permission to use hypnosis with a child (Wester, 2013). These releases or consent forms are either sent ahead of time or presented at the initial appointment. I don't do this for a few reasons. First, my goal is to normalize the use of hypnosis as a part of what I will do with a child. Is it special? Different? A new experience for many? Sure. But a separate consent form sends the message that it is too distinct, and in my opinion suggests the negative connotations of hypnosis that impede wider acceptance. Parents provide consent to treatment and I consider hypnosis as part of that treatment. Second, I want the exchange of questions and information to be part of a face-to-face conversation. This contact matters because it is an opportunity to build rapport and interact in a way that may influence the intervention, which I discuss in detail in Chapter 3. Finally, it gives me more flexibility in how and when I introduce hypnosis.

THE PATH YOU'RE TAKING, THE SEEDS I'M PLANTING

This book is designed to be a practical guide, as if you and I were sitting together and you said to me, "Hey, Lynn, I'm working with children who [fill in the blank] and I'd like to use hypnosis. Do you have any ideas?" My intent is to provide you with the structure and techniques to create effective hypnosis sessions, and to offer plentiful ideas, words, and examples to launch your own creativity and language.

Chapter 2 addresses logistical and frequently asked questions regarding the use of scripts, issues of responsiveness, and the important role of childhood development in your interventions. Chapter 3 helps you capitalize on those important first contacts with children and parents. What can you notice and what seeds can you plant that will build momentum in the direction of change?

Chapter 4 describes how to identify what a child and family need and then offer helpful new frameworks, perspectives, and skills using hypnotic strategies. This chapter answers the important questions: How do I figure out what to say in a hypnosis session? How can I target my interventions most effectively? Chapter 5 then offers a template for delivering the session, moving you sequentially through each element of a session and helping you create a compelling experience such that the new frame is accepted and absorbed.

Chapters 6, 7, 8, and 9 get specific, helping you take what you've learned in the previous chapters and apply it to the specific (but often overlapping) problems that clinicians and health care providers most often treat: anxiety, depression, medical issues such as pain, illness, and procedures, and sleep issues.

Chapter 10 talks specifically about the role of parents. When do you include them? How can they help? What can you offer to parents that will enhance the family's success? How can you use hypnosis to help with parenting and connection?

Chapter 11 addresses the larger issues and some of the challenges of incorporating pediatric hypnosis into the treatment of children and families. Consider it my final opportunity to make a case for the joyful use of this effective tool, a not-so-subtle suggestion to absorb yourself in the playfulness of words, metaphors, and curiosity.

I hope that as you move through the chapters, you'll consistently imagine how to incorporate my words into your own practice and style, and grow increasingly excited and confident about the rich opportunities to use hypnosis, formally and informally, to create positive experiences and frameworks for the families you meet.

CHAPTER *2*

Concrete Considerations

Responsiveness, Scripts,
and the Role of Development

*G*etting better at hypnosis (or guitar or swimming or long divi-
sion) requires practicing and doing. Improving your ability to offer
a transformative experience to a child requires, of course, that you
actually offer the experience. As the Russian physician and writer
Anton Chekhov said, "Knowledge is of no value unless you put it
into practice."

This is, above all, a book about doing hypnosis. Nonetheless, before we dive into the doing, a few topics are worth covering
upfront as they will inform the doing to come. These topics include
hypnotic responsiveness in children, the use of suggestibility tests
and scripts, and the influence of child development on your hypnotic
interventions.

ASSESSING HYPNOTIC RESPONSIVENESS: WHAT DO WE KNOW AND WHAT DO WE NEED TO KNOW?

There is a long-held consensus (or perhaps more of an accepted belief) among researchers and clinicians that children are more hypnotizable than adults, with the peak responsiveness during preadolescence (see e.g., Morgan & Hilgard, 1978; Olness & Gardner, 1988; Plotnick & O'Grady, 1991). However, when you begin to look at the many unanswered questions and difficulties inherent in measuring children's hypnotic responsiveness, it's not that definitive. In fact, because hypnosis with children often looks different from what most people imagine it to be, the basic question arises whether or not it's truly hypnosis. This question is no less complex when it comes to adults, based on the multiple theories and concepts about what hypnosis is and why it works. For a clear summary of the different perspectives and further resources, see *Trancework* by Yapko (2012, Chapter 3), and discussions by Lynn (Lynn, Vanderhoff, Shindler, & Stafford, 2002; Lynn et al., 2005; Lynn, 2007), Kirsch (1994), and Chaves (1997, 1999).

I offer you a few examples of the many interesting questions researchers have posed about children and responsiveness. LeBaron (1983) examined the relationship between a child's responsiveness and the role of fantasy in the family, but found that many other factors were most likely at play. London (1962) also questioned susceptibility as a function of a child's relationships to parental figures and other personality traits. Vandenberg (2002) questioned the tests that showed low responsiveness in children under 7 years old, because clinical evidence and reporting seemed to suggest otherwise. He concluded that younger children experience hypnosis differently than older children due to their level of cognitive development and executive functioning. (I address this issue in more detail in the next section.)

Kohen and Olness did a marvelous job of looking at the past and current research, examining the many studies that attempt to weed out the factors that influence a child's hypnotic responsiveness, and came to this conclusion: "The truth is that we really cannot say very much with confidence concerning hypnotic responsiveness in children" (2011, p. 33).

What does this mean for clinicians working to provide assistance to children in need of help? That we must have developmental knowledge and awareness of ongoing research, but ultimately the child in front of us, our communication with the child, and whether or not we're helping the child will best guide our interventions.

SUGGESTIBILITY TESTS

The Stanford Hypnotic Clinical Scale for Children (Morgan & Hilgard, 1978) and the Children's Hypnotic Susceptibility Scale (London, 1962) were designed to measure a child's hypnotic responsiveness on a variety of scales, and have been used to compare broader patterns of responsiveness between children of different ages and between children and adults. The tests generally consist of a brief induction (eye closure and then staring or relaxing for older children and suggestions of pretending or imagining for younger children) followed by measurement of performance on various hypnotic phenomena, such as hand lowering, age regression, and auditory and visual hallucination.

I do not use formal suggestibility tests in my clinical practice, and I can honestly say that I don't know any other practicing clinicians that use them regularly or formally with children in their clinical practices.

That said, collaboratively using a scale with a child or teen can enhance treatment in some circumstances. First, it's a way to introduce hypnosis without any performance pressure, perhaps demystifying it for both child and parents. Older children and teens may be curious at best (and suspicious at worst) about what you're going to "make them do," so they can experience this trial run as casual and educational. Fourteen-year-old Greta came to see me to address her fear of flying. She wanted to use hypnosis but had recently seen a hypnosis show at a fair, and was worried about what I would say and how she would perform. I told her that hypnosis was a way to use her imagination to learn new things or practice different experiences, and that going inside and pretending could change how her mind and body react to things.

> *For example, close your eyes for a moment . . . and hold out your left arm in front of you, straight and with the palm up. Now imagine I'm putting a rock into your hand. . . . Feel the rock in your fingers. . . . It's fairly heavy . . . and just imagine your arm and hand responding to that heavy rock. . . . Can you feel it? . . . It may feel a little heavier . . . or maybe a lot heavier. . . . Just imagine . . .*

Her arm slowly dropped, and when we finished and she opened her eyes, I said, "That's a way to see how you respond. . . . You did so well on that I think we can use it again when we do the hypnosis."

And what if Greta hadn't responded? I would first ask her what she was experiencing, because, although her arm didn't move as far as I could see, she could surprise me and say, "I could feel the rock and my arm floating down. . . . It was cool!" If she confirmed what I was seeing (no response), I might then ask her what she was experiencing and build upon that. Did it feel like her arm was lighter instead of heavier? Interesting! Or I might wonder with her what sensations she could imagine creating. . . . Heat? Coolness? Lightness? What if she refused to participate or said she felt nothing? That would offer me important information, perhaps about her willingness (or unwillingness) to respond to direct suggestions, and I might amplify the skill of being able to "feel nothing at the right times to feel nothing" as a way to help her manage the airplane flight.

Such information is helpful as you introduce the process of hypnosis, while staying a few steps away from the specific content of the child's issue. Playing with creating hypnotic phenomena in this nonthreatening way can build rapport and enhance both a sense of mastery and positive anticipation of what's to come (Gfeller & Gorassini, 2010; Lynn & Kirsch, 2006; Kirsch, 1985). It also presents an opportunity to make indirect suggestions that pave the way for your work together, what Michael Yapko (2006) termed the "pre-work work." Why miss the chance to suggest, for example, how "the ability to create different responses in your mind and in your body can be a cool thing to discover about yourself"?

Assessing a child's skill or preference for certain hypnotic phenomena may also give you, the clinician, help in identifying the type of suggestions that best fit a particular child. After experimenting with the inductions on the scale, you both may discover, for example, that your 10-year-old client does quite well with visual hallucination or suggestions but lousy with auditory hallucination. Therefore, as you are helping him prepare for his dental procedure, together you create a plan that plays to his strengths and builds on his confidence, suggesting:

We discovered sitting here together how great you are at seeing things in your imagination . . . even with your eyes closed . . . and when you're sitting in Dr. Walker's chair . . . you can see the bright light shining through your eyelids . . . which can remind you of that great memory of the lights at Fenway [a baseball stadium] . . . shining so brightly. . . . When you went to the night game last month with your dad . . . you were able to tell me so many details . . . and you can surround yourself right now in the sights you see . . . the green field . . . the white bases . . . all the red hats in the crowd . . . and while the dentist works on your mouth out here . . . you can see yourself smiling on the inside . . . as you imagine and remember . . . .

SCRIPTS

Many hypnosis books, certifications, and training courses offer standardized written scripts to participants and little else. This unfortunately promotes the idea that hypnosis is simply the act of reading words and suggestions from the right script; such limited training also negates the importance of interacting creatively and flexibly with both children and adults. Prefabricated scripts designed for particular problems—like anxiety or sleep or focus or weight—miss the point, namely that the hypnotic experience you offer to a child should be collaborative and custom fit, and that the solutions, when we engage and lead, often come from the child. Pulling out a written script and reading it to the person in front you is sometimes accepted (and expected) by adults (although I don't and don't want you to either), but it's impossible for me to imagine how this could work in an interactive encounter with a child.

This does not mean you shouldn't use and adapt other people's words and ideas, as they can be helpful and inspiring. Did you come across a great metaphor? Use it! Is there a theme or phrase or approach that might work with your client? Try it! I want the examples in this book to get your own imagination going and to provide guidance if you're new to hypnosis and looking to build confidence. But I do not recommend reading scripts aloud (including ones you write yourself) to a client of any age, even as a beginner. Go ahead and feel awkward as you learn to assess, target, create, and deliver. This book is designed to help with this process of trying it out. In my opinion, the crutch of a prewritten script will only impede your learning and take your focus off the child sitting in front of you.

This no-script instruction, which I strongly recommend to you, requires a bit of a caveat. While I implore you to avoid reading scripts, I often use illustrated books in my office. As a follow-up assignment, I recommend that parents and children read particular storybooks that promote the new cognitive responses and frameworks that I'm simultaneously suggesting in our therapy together. Many children and parents enjoy the ritual of sharing a book, with its time for closeness, looking at the illustrations, and even turning the pages. Older children may prefer to read on their own. Either way, a well-chosen book becomes an entrancing adjunct to the process of therapeutic change.

Metaphor and storytelling are integral to the hypnotic process and to learning in general (Burns, 2005, 2007; Thomson, 2005, 2009; Linden, 2003; Erickson & Rossi, 1979). I suggest that you explore children's books and create your own collection that addresses common themes. Throughout the upcoming chapters, I incorporate and recommend children's literature as a way to enhance suggestions. You'll find an annotated list of great children's books in Appendix B to get you started.

DEVELOPMENT AND ITS ROLE IN HYPNOSIS WITH CHILDREN

How does hypnosis with children differ from that with adults? How can we best adapt adult approaches to the children we see in our practices? How do I approach a 6-year-old with asthma differently than a 12-year-old?

Understanding and then harnessing the developmental abilities of children and teens will make your interventions better. You must join this knowledge, however, with the larger goal of "being attuned to the child's whole being, his or her world, and the unique nature of his or her difficulty" (Kuttner & Catchpole, 2013, p. 26). I can recall two children of about the same age (5) working on the issue of bedwetting. One child was thrilled with the idea of sending messages between his brain and bladder and decided to use a speedy rocket; the other, when offered a similar idea of sending messages, said, "Bladders don't talk, Lynn. Let's be real."

Early Childhood (Approximately 3–7)

Children between the ages of 3 and 7 are said to be in the early childhood or preoperational phase, according to Piaget's (1962) framework of development. Although this is defined as a single stage by Piaget, huge changes occur in cognitive and emotional development during these years. Wall (1991) pointed out that from start to finish of this phase, children move from very low hypnotizability into the age range most often viewed as the peak of hypnotizability. For example, changes in the perception of time, the ability to understand metaphor, and even the willingness for eye closure happen between 4 and 7. Therefore, I repeat: it is most important to pay attention to the child in front of you, guided by your observations and the child's feedback.

Imagination and magical thinking are prominent, with easy and frequent movement between fantasy and reality. Children learn much through their play, which is active and externally focused. Critical to this period is the seeking of mastery and competence through what Italian educator Maria Montessori (1966) referred to as "work," or a creative interaction with the environment. Erik Erikson (1959) defined this as the "industry" stage: the age of doing, full of pretending, role-playing, and making stuff. Children often begin school and move from a more passive relationship with the world toward a realization that they can actively influence outcomes.

They have little ability to go inside and imagine; their busy imaginations are externally represented and acted out with roles, games, props, and puppets (Kuttner & Catchpole, 2013). A 4-year-old doesn't want to just think about being a firefighter in his head; he wants to be a firefighter, with a truck made of boxes, a pot for a helmet, and lots of loud sirens of his own creation. Games and fantasies allow for the development of new skills. Aamodt and Wang said it well: "An average four-year-old child who is asked to stand still for as long as possible can manage it for slightly less than one minute.

If he's asked to pretend he's a guard outside a castle, though, he can hold his pose four times as long" (2011, p. 117).

Young children mainly live in the present. They do not think too far into the future or have an accurate understanding of time. They may understand "before" and "after," but don't know the difference between yesterday and two weeks ago, or tomorrow and next month. Any parent of a 4- or 5-year-old knows that announcing plans for a fun trip that's weeks or months away results in daily questioning and urgency, as if the trip were happening tomorrow. Suggesting to a 6-year-old that he imagine how he'll feel comfortable in the future when he adjusts to kindergarten won't work. Helping him practice and plan for tomorrow morning would be a more effective approach, with self-hypnosis or role-playing tasks (cued by an adult) to help him feel in charge of his morning:

MOM (at bedtime): So this is Tuesday night, and tomorrow is Wednesday morning, a school morning, right? So let's pretend it's the morning and I come in to wake you up. Let's imagine together. Good morning! Rise and shine!

JAMES: Good morning . . .

MOM: Now let's imagine the three things you do to get ready for your day. . . . What's the first one?

JAMES: I have to get ready with clothes and breakfast.

MOM: Right. . . . You did it today . . . remember? Tomorrow will feel easier because you know what to do. . . . Now what comes next?

Hypnosis with children in this stage is a fluid and interactive experience. Asking a young child to close his eyes, sit quietly, and imagine something internally is rarely successful. In fact, Morgan and Hilgard (1978) found that while most children age 8 and over responded to a permissive suggestion for eye closure, none under the age of 5 did so. Age regression or suggestions that ask a child to pretend to dream or "imagine that you're dreaming" are too cogni-tively complex (Vandenberg, 2002). After the age of 4, the ability to connect the past with present events appears, although for 4-year-olds, memory is fragile and easily influenced by adults (Kagan, 2013).

On the other hand, I routinely see children this age become deeply absorbed in a hypnotic experience, as long as there is a focus on play, pretending, and often some external cueing. Children are often happy to create and accept irrational explanations, allowing for solutions that are free of real-world limitations. At this age, we can make magical suggestions, or simply enjoy and elaborate upon what the child offers. Preschoolers will participate in the telling of a story in a way that absorbs and dissociates them (helpful for medical settings) or create characters that join the child in the solution of a problem or the development of ego strength (Kuttner, 1988; Linden, 2003; Tilton, 1984). Five-year-olds are beginning to understand the difference between real and imaginary, but still move easily between the two. This free use of magic gives children the ability to feel effec-tive. As Linden wrote, "Children understand magic as a way to make things happen that ordinarily cannot happen. It can give children a sense of control and mastery in situations which seem hopeless, and does so with delight and joy" (2003, p. 247).

For example, Lucy was almost 5 when her parents separated. When she transitioned between the two houses, she often cried for hours and had great difficulty falling asleep for the first night or two in either house. Lucy's parents said all the right things. They explained to Lucy that she had two houses now and that both par-ents loved her all the time, no matter which house she was in. When Lucy told me she had "two houses but only one dog" (and the dog, Blue, did not travel between the two houses), I suggested we come up with a plan to help her feel connected to her dog when she was away from him. Lucy decided that Blue needed a message from her every day when she was gone. We got several envelopes and little pieces of paper, and wrote simple messages to Blue. "I'll leave the messages for Blue and he will read them every day I'm gone," Lucy said.

"And you will know he is reading them," I said, "because when you get back to Dad's house, and he wags his tail and licks you, you will hear him saying thank you in doggy talk. And he will think of you when you're not there, and you will think of him, and when he reads your messages you'll be connected like magic."

Middle Childhood (Ages 7–11)

I overheard a conversation between two friends recently. Both have children around 3 or 4 years old, one with a set of twins. They were relating recent tales of illogical battles over socks and vegetables and the acceptable colors of plastic cups. "We just have to hang in there," one said to the other. "My sister-in-law told me that something changes when they turn 7."

Ah, the concrete operational period. Latency. The phase when parents notice a shift in their child's ability to cooperate, manage tasks more independently, and see themselves as a member of a cooperative group. As I said earlier, great changes occur in children cognitively, emotionally, and socially as they approach age 7. Vandenberg (2002) referred to this as a "watershed" in human development when children become aware of their own thoughts and aware that others have thoughts and feelings different from their own.

Jerome Kagan (2013), the distinguished developmental psychologist, described some of the emerging developments in 7-year-olds: they can distinguish between events that will happen further in the future versus those that will occur more immediately, can use past experiences to both anticipate the difficulty of a task and activate strategies to improve performance, and show an emerging ability to see different perspectives of the same event.

A school psychologist and friend of mine who works with elementary school kids describes them as willing to take risks without the self-consciousness of older children. From her observations, they remain fairly self-oriented, but love to engage with others. They begin to notice the world around them and come up with interesting perspectives and views of their environment, including some amusing conclusions about the adults around them. Again, we see the burgeoning ability to step outside of one's own experience (Julie Bassi, PhD, personal communication, 2013).

Children in this phase are still concrete in their thinking, but are developing the ability to solve problems with logic. They are beginning, with coaching, to make more sophisticated connections and comparisons, for example, transferring learning from one context to other contexts (Bransford, Brown, & Cocking, 2000). Thus, they are able to use metaphor, but often need guidance in making the connections between the metaphor, themselves, and the desired outcome (Wall, 1991). This is the stage where it's likely important to help with connections by saying something like, "I'm telling you this story about X because it relates to you in this way." In fact, it's important to remember that concrete thinkers, no matter what age or stage, often benefit from this kind of framing of stories and metaphors to help make a therapeutic point (Yapko, 1983, 2012).

Amid all the blossoming of these new and more sophisticated ways of thinking, children in this stage are still happily willing to be freely imaginative. They are more able to close their eyes and imagine internally, without the props and activity of younger children, although in my experience eyes will open and close throughout the interaction. In fact, Cooper and London (1976) found that children between 7 and 11 were more alert when eyes were closed than open, based on EEG readings. (So what do we say about eye closure? It varies.)

At this stage children will "float away on a cloud" or "imagine hitting a home run to win the game." They are more willing to transport themselves internally to that experience and become entranced by it. They are capable of taking what they practice in a session with the therapist and then using it more independently to create their own experience of "self-hypnosis" (Kuttner & Catchpole, 2013, p. 38). As mentioned in Chapter 1, I routinely record sessions for children to listen to later as a way to practice their skills. Ultimately they move away from using the recording, internalizing what we did together and making it their own.

Seven-year-old Robert came to see me because he was anxious about "having a poop accident on the bus" on the way to school. His morning routine had become extremely focused on using the bathroom repeatedly. He refused to eat breakfast, and falling asleep at night was getting difficult as he anticipated waking for school the next morning. After a complete medical workup that found no physical issues, we began talking together about Robert's Worry. Then we externalized it and began talking directly to it: "You only show up on school nights," Robert said. He grabbed a piece of paper and told me he was going to draw what was happening. "My amygdala [we had gone over pictures of the brain and Robert understood that his amygdala was his brain's alarm center] stays in my brain over the weekend, but on school nights he moves down into my poop shoot," Robert said, drawing his version of the amygdala moving from his head to his gut. "I need to stop Worry from sending my amygdala down there." This led to regular role-playing, first with me and then his parents playing the role of Worry while Robert took charge. He often used a paper and pen to diagram what was happening in his body and how he was going to change it, explaining and imagining as he drew, "I just have to put my amygdala back where it belongs."

Robert's story illustrates the seamless combination of real and imaginary worlds. Robert understands the mind-body connection and how his thinking creates bodily responses. He grasps the concept of cause and effect. But he also accepts and enjoys the fact that his solutions don't need to follow the rules of anatomy.

Adolescence and Beyond

As much as the latency stage gets parental acclaim for its relative ease, adolescence has a reputation that routinely evokes rolling of the eyes or predictions of doom. Our society often views people who work (by choice) at middle schools with a combination of reverence and disbelief, as if these people willingly opt to handle nuclear waste. Clearly parents are working to understand the teen brain. I did a Google search with the phrase "understanding your teen" and it came back with 35,600,000 hits. Amazon showed over 3,700 titles when I searched the subject "parenting teens."

With so many resources exploring and explaining the breadth of the adolescent journey, I focus here on the developmental considerations that will most impact and elevate your use of hypnosis with teens.

To remain consistent, let's first look at Piaget's conception of adolescent cognitive development, defined as the formal operational stage. This stage is marked by the increased ability to think abstractly, make connections between specific individual experiences and the experiences of others, and regulate and use one's own cognitive strategies, broadly referred to as metacognition (Brown, 1987). Studies indicate that metacognitive ability is present during middle childhood, improves across the period of adolescence, peaks in late adolescence, and then stabilizes in adulthood (Weil et al., 2013).

The development of more abstract and sophisticated thinking means that the language used during hypnosis can be both direct and indirect (based on the individual) and more similar to what we do with adults. Teens can understand and create metaphors and now have the ability to think about hypothetical situations that they have never experienced (Kagan, 2013). Adolescents also discover hypocrisy in others and cognitive dissonance in themselves, as they try to create what Kagan (2013, p. 153) called a "semantic consistency" between what they see in others, what they feel in themselves, and what they believe to be moral or immoral.

Adolescents are famously in the process of creating their own identity and self-concept (Sebastian, Burnett, & Blakemore, 2008). Erik Erikson (1959) referred to the conflict of this stage as identity versus confusion; the core of adolescent turmoil is often described as the push-pull conflict teens have with adults as they seek to discover what they and their futures will look like (Klimstra, 2013; Wiley & Berman, 2013). In terms of brain development, adolescents experience major reorganization, resulting in desires for more novelty and increased social connection. They also tend to underestimate the consequences of their actions (Aamodt & Wang, 2011).

Two popular books on parenting teens address adolescence with both insight and respect. Anthony Wolf's *Get Out of My Life, but First Can You Drive Me and Cheryl to the Mall?* described the developmental mandate that "tells the adolescent to turn away from childhood and childish feelings," which means they must turn away from their parents in order to develop their autonomy (2002, pp. 14–15).

Michael Riera, author of *Staying Connected to Your Teenager*, saw the concept of separation and independence as both outdated and inaccurate. Instead he supported a more successful "concept of extension," where teens must venture out and extend away from their parents, while parents need to remain connected (in a different way compared to childhood) to their teen during this time of change and vulnerability (Riera, 2003, p. 4).

How do new cognitive abilities and intense developmental conflict impact your hypnotic interventions with teens? Here's my bias: it creates exciting options and challenges. Think about it: here's a person who is busy inside, with thoughts and ideas, who seeks novelty and connection, and whose pursuit of independence and mastery is now a full-time job, developmentally speaking. And although a teen can potentially be more self-conscious and thus initially less willing to put himself into this new situation of hypnosis (and more aware of the myths and connotations that come along with using the word *hypnosis*), many teens and young adults see this as an opportunity to try something interesting, even cool. Oftentimes, the teens that come to see me for therapy—and are less than excited about the prospect of talking to a stranger about their problems—are intrigued by the idea of experiencing hypnosis. They are curious about an experience that fits many of their adolescent criteria: a combination of mastery, creativity, newness, and connection to the clinician.

Because this is such a time of change, teens often present with complicated and overwhelming issues. The ability to sort through and prioritize the many factors at play is both a critical component in the development of your intervention and a skill you want to model for your maturing client. (Chapter 4 discusses in detail how to best target and create your interventions.) An early hypnosis session that focuses on how to organize and prioritize life's challenges offers an overwhelmed teen an experience that introduces this skill on multiple levels and sets the stage for the work to come. Rather than spend time talking about what's overwhelming, use hypnosis to experientially model taking action while creating an alliance that builds trust (Yapko, 2012; Gfeller & Gorassini, 2010).

Tanya came to see me when she was 16. A lot was happening in her life, including her father's remarriage and his planned move to another state, her first boyfriend of any importance, and the beginning of college discussions at her high school. Her mother insisted she see a therapist after noticing superficial scratches on her arms and Tanya's subsequent confession that she was up at night worrying about all that was in front of her.

Tanya's description of her current circumstances and the worry that came with it was tangled and messy—for both of us. I suggested she might like an opportunity to settle back for a few minutes and get a bit of distance from all that was swirling around her:

> *If you'd like, you can close your eyes and just enjoy the feel of gravity pulling you gently into the cushions of the couch. . . . You can slow down for a bit . . . because you certainly have so much going on . . . and you might be tired of hearing it from adults . . . but you are in a time of transition, of figuring out what's growing stronger . . . and what you're ready to leave behind . . . your friendships, your family, your physical body, even the way you think and understand things. . . . They're shifting and changing. . . . It's like deciding to redecorate your room . . . and you have to start somewhere . . . but there are so many possible paint colors to choose from . . . and so many rugs . . . and maybe that bed isn't too small just yet . . . but slowly you move forward, choice by choice, breaking it down . . . feeling excited and unsure at the same time . . . figuring out what you'll change and what can stay the same for now . . . and imagining what the final product might be, but not knowing for sure. . . . And you've taken some important steps . . . like asking for advice. . . . As a Chinese philosopher said . . . "The journey of a thousand miles begins with a single step" . . . or as my little niece reminded me . . . the only way to eat a moose is . . . one bite at a time.*

An important theme in this short intervention was Tanya's recognition that she was moving ahead into uncertainty without knowing exactly how to do it all, but that she would take steps and have guidance along the way (as she was doing in that moment with me).

And this compels me to highlight one more factor before we leave this discussion of development and hypnosis: the importance of social interaction and the value of connection when using hypnosis at all levels of development.

31

HYPNOSIS AND DEVELOPMENT:
MORE THAN THE SUM OF THEIR PARTS

While we certainly want to match our interventions to the developmental capabilities of the child, I also find it exciting to think about hypnosis as a way to lead children along, to invite them into an experience they didn't know they were capable of having, and even creating solutions that might, at first blush, seem too advanced or challenging. Lev Vygotsky, a Russian psychologist who died in 1934, described the "zone of proximal development," a place where functions are in the process of maturing but not yet fully developed, where the skills are buds or flowers of development rather than fruit (Vygotsky, 1997). Stressing the importance of social interaction, he believed it limiting to look only at development based on what a child can do alone, but instead looked at what a child achieves through problem solving while collaborating with more capable peers or under adult guidance (Vygotsky, 1997). The social connection of hypnosis—the support that a child and her parents feel when we connect to them and show them what's possible—perhaps taps into this zone. Maybe this is why clinicians experience so profoundly what sometimes research alone fails to convey about the success of pediatric hypnosis (Milling & Costantino, 2000) and why Kohen and Olness's (2011) conclusion that most studies underestimate the hypnotic capabilities of children rings so true.

CHAPTER *3*

The Initial Contact

Amplifying the Benefits of Hypnotic Communication Right From the Start

*B*ased on how difficult it is to define hypnosis with children, it's even trickier (and perhaps unnecessary) if we feel the need to pinpoint exactly when and how we start using hypnosis with kids. My response to this frequently asked question? Immediately. From the start, we can invite children to participate in change, and when they accept our invitation, they become willing participants in what happens next. Zeig (2006, p. 115) used the analogy of a legal contract: the therapist "applies for the right to influence," and the client agrees by responding to the cues and suggestions of the therapist. Consider this my invitation to you to take what you already know as a clinician and start to enhance it with hypnotic processes.

Whether or not you introduce hypnosis formally or informally depends on the expectations, age, and circumstances of the child and parents. In some circumstances, the child and parents may be seeking out hypnosis. They expect a distinct experience with a formal invitation to shift attention, change body position, and often close their eyes. This can be helpful, because defining the situation as hypnosis can improve responsiveness to suggestions (Kirsch, 1985; Sliwinski & Elkins, 2013). For example, as I said in Chapter 2, teens in particular may perceive hypnosis as different from therapy and be more willing to engage. Capitalizing on the positive expectations that the term *hypnosis* creates for some improves outcomes (Kirsch, 1985).

Often, however, children and parents come to see me for therapy, not necessarily hypnosis. There may be no stated expectation that we will be doing hypnosis together. In medical or other settings, psychotherapy or hypnosis is not the purpose of the visit or contact at all. My own understanding of when we start doing hypnosis with children relies on these four premises:

1. Hypnotic phenomena are ever present in our encounters with children.
2. Our goal is to use these hypnotic tools and moments in versatile ways that best fit the person in front of us.
3. Great interventions build, layer upon layer from the ground up.
4. We should focus on the creating and/or supporting of positive resources.

Regardless of the circumstances or setting of the initial meeting with a child, "hypnosis happens," and therefore recognizing and capturing these hypnotic opportunities from the start creates the opportunity to shift a child's perceptions of his world and himself in a positive way (Berberich, 2007).

In this chapter I explain how to better think, plan, and interact in a hypnotic or suggestive way from the very first contact. How can you use these first valuable minutes to lay the important groundwork of connection and change, even before you fully know what's going on with the child and what your treatment will look like? Your introduction to the particular content of a child's issues may be straightforward and concrete, or unique and overwhelming. You may hear different information from different parents, or meet a child who behaves and reacts nothing like the parents predicted. No matter what you encounter, the challenge—and the fun—of using hypnosis more effectively is when, from the start, you strategically begin to till the soil of change even as you are still determining what seeds to plant and where to plant them (Zeig, 1980, 1988).

Jay Haley's description of Erickson's use of seeding in *Uncommon Therapy* inspires us to be strategic and purposeful from the start: "With families, Erickson will introduce, or emphasize, certain ideas in the beginning of the interchange, so that later, if he wants to achieve a certain response, he has already laid the groundwork for that response" (1973, p. 34). Seeds are planted early based on your recognition of common themes and patterns and your observations of this particular family.

WHOM TO SEE FIRST?

People often ask me if I see the child alone, the parents alone, or the child and parent together. In general, I want the parents and the child there at the first meeting. I may ask the parents to go to the waiting room, or the child to leave for a bit. I have no hard and fast rule, and I urge you to be flexible, too. Utilize. Be creative. Be aware of the many options and use them flexibly. Be the chess player who sees the whole board. Different combinations and dynamics of family members in the treatment room reveal interesting information.

I talk more about the role of parents during hypnosis in Chapter 10. In general, most experts agree that autonomy and mastery are important pieces of the experience, and that overinvolvement by parents is detrimental (Gardner, 1974b; Kohen, Olness, Colwell, &

Heimel, 1984). In my experience, rapport can be greatly enhanced when parents are given information, allowed to observe when appropriate, and are offered their own opportunity to have a hypnotic experience separate from their child. I also have had success when together we come up with a collaborative approach that allows a parent to be a helper or assistant when needed. Again, my emphasis is on flexible guidelines that are adapted to best build cooperation and curiosity.

I generally do a 90-minute first session because I have the flexibility to do that. Different treatment settings have different restrictions. I'm aware of the rules that psychotherapy and other settings impose. Some of them don't work for me, and they don't work for the children and families I see.

Circumstances sometimes exist where having information about a child prior to the first interview is necessary. Parents may wish to talk openly with you about the struggles they are having with their child but do not wish the child to be a part of this difficult conversation. Family circumstances, medical history, marital issues, or other topics may not be appropriate for the child to hear. Meeting alone with the parents prior to meeting with the child can be helpful both to exchange this information and because of what you will learn about the parents' frames of reference and their unedited view of the problem. I've had many parent interviews where the problem is described in catastrophic terms, with tired parents predicting a complete and utter lack of cooperation by their child upon meeting me. Then, despite their dire predictions, the child arrives eager to talk openly about her struggles. This is interesting information. Keep in mind that even these parent-only assessments allow for suggestions that may shift frameworks and anticipate future interactions.

If the primary client is an adolescent, she can and should contribute valuable information to the history taking. Her description of her situation (and how she presents herself out of the presence of family members) helps to develop a framework of the problem and the potential solutions, a framework that may be very different than the one portrayed by one or more of the parents.

Reports from school, including testing and other diagnostic information, can be helpful, but consider seeing the child first to observe and interact with her free of others' opinions. The exception is any kind of issue that impacts your ability to communicate effectively, such as a hearing impairment or cognitive delay.

Parents may also choose to e-mail you a history of the problem and their experiences treating it. This can work well, so that a child's first session is not filled with history taking and discussion of past failures. Even so, there are times when hearing face to face how a family describes what didn't work and why past efforts have fallen short is also illuminating. I'll be more specific about how to use past history positively in your initial meeting later in the chapter when I talk about accessing resources.

My own guideline: I gather history ahead of time from parents (optimally in person) if I suspect that such information is extensive, negative, or urgent enough that I'll be unable to get a solid clinical picture without it. I also may choose to talk to the parents first if their agenda differs from the child's, or if information about a child's perception of the problem or resistance to treatment is best known ahead of time. This allows me to plan ahead a bit (so as not to be caught too off guard) and successfully focus my intervention on the child sitting in front of me.

The story of Amy illustrates the benefit of meeting with parents ahead of time. Her parents requested we meet alone first because 9-year-old Amy was very resistant to seeing a therapist, but agreed to come only if we focused on her agenda: Amy had a fear of dogs that she wanted to get rid of, because—despite her fear—she badly wanted a dog of her own. Her parents were much more concerned about their daughter's pervasive inability to manage any type of change or surprise in the routine of school or home. She had already been to two therapists, but whenever her parents or the therapist tried to talk about her sporadic refusal to attend school or her frequent tantrums when plans didn't go as she expected, she became angry and silent. Because she was unwilling to talk about her parents' concerns and refusing to participate in the therapy in any way, the sessions quickly ended.

Because I knew this ahead of time, I focused only on the dog issue in the first session, planting seeds along the way about fears, surprises, and the unpredictability of dogs and puppies. This was safe territory that allowed me to build rapport, show her I was listening to her wants, and suggest movement toward a new, more malleable framework. Amy's dog phobia subsided after three or four sessions. (I talk about using hypnosis with anxiety in Chapter 6.) I was then able to move into the touchier topic of her school refusal and anxiety, using the success she had with dogs—and her trust in me—to ease the transition.

As I said above, each initial meeting is an opportunity to connect and learn and intervene. Let's now look at three important—and very intertwined—components of the initial contact or interview:

1. Building rapport
2. Observation of key elements and patterns in the child and other family members
3. Deliberate use of language and suggestion

Certainly these components are not as distinct as a numbered list implies; they weave through your initial interview and are part of your ongoing contact with a child. Even describing them as distinct from each other becomes a challenge because ideally you are simultaneously building rapport, observing, and communicating with a family. Nor are these three components the exclusive domain of hypnosis. But let's capitalize on the versatility of hypnotic suggestion to bolster your treatment by creating positive momentum quickly. During the first meeting, even the first phone contact, you can begin to predict, encourage, and augment positive change.

BUILDING RAPPORT

Have you ever called technical support because your computer has crashed and the support person on the phone starts with a polite request to "make sure your computer is plugged in and turned on"? For me, discussing the importance of building rapport, particularly with children, feels as obvious. Of course we need to build rapport. Connecting with a child and her parents creates trust and collaboration. Listening attentively, reflecting back the family's concerns, and expressing your own optimism about reducing the family's struggle allow them to settle into the experiences to come.

Someone who is "good with kids" gets down on the floor with a toddler and also knows how to respectfully listen to the social complexities of being a teenager. Someone who connects with children talks directly at their level of understanding without condescension. Being fluent in the developmental stages of children in a general way while appreciating the specific needs of the child in front of you is a given, as discussed in Chapter 2.

Connecting with children comes easier to some than to others. Knowing your own predilections, preferences, and abilities to relate to children in different age groups—or to children at all—is critically important. And this is not to say such abilities are static. As your life and life experiences change, your abilities to better relate to those in a particular age group may improve or wither. Pay attention to this. If the match is not there, sometimes it's much better for the client, and ultimately you, to steer him toward a therapist who may be a good, perhaps even great, match. I have a colleague who performs an initial interview, not so much to determine whether the family will continue to seek counseling from the therapist, but rather for the therapist to determine if the match will allow him to do effective therapy.

Giving your attention and respect to a child when you first meet creates a level of trust that is necessary when stepping into a child's personal experience. My family dentist manages this successfully in a tricky setting with his clear "no parents in the treatment room" policy. Parents are informed of what's to come. They give their consent and are left in the waiting area. When the dental assistant and the dentist address children at their level, with honesty and warmth, the majority of the patients do fine without their parents. (He would say they do better without the parents.) When a child is in the presence of someone completely focused and listening intently, the message is clear: "I am paying attention and working to understand what you are experiencing in this situation. And I know what I'm doing." Their focus and experienced confidence are contagious—as contagious as the focused worry of a parent in the waiting room, they would surely tell you.

Does my dentist know that he's using hypnotic techniques to manage his young patients' fear? I doubt it. But here's what he exemplifies: when we aim to enhance responsiveness, we want to build rapport in a deliberate way that first lets the child know we understand, and then facilitates the acceptance of suggestions to follow (Lynn & Kirsch, 2006; Zeig, 1990, 2001; Sliwinski & Elkins, 2013). Erickson and Rossi said it well: "Acknowledging the patient's current reality thus opens a yes set for whatever suggestions the therapist may wish to introduce" (1979, p. 5).

The goal, then, is to be fully present and acknowledge what's happening with the child, while suggesting (and demonstrating) where you are headed and how you can help. The sooner you connect with the child, the sooner you begin to shift her toward a solution. My dentist wouldn't describe his approach as creating a yes set that allows for more cooperation and easier treatment. Perhaps he'd call it hypnotic. Whatever the terminology, he's skilled at building rapport with positive suggestions and focus in a way that moves his treatment forward.

Sugarman and Wester (2013) describe the effective process of pacing and leading, using pacing to acknowledge empathically where the child is at the present moment ("You don't look too happy to be here today") and using leading to suggest the possibility of change ("But maybe you'll feel differently by the time you head out the door"). Think for a moment about someone in your life who did or didn't use this well and the impact on you. I remember being a squeamish child getting a shot from a gruff nurse who said, "There's no reason to cry. This won't hurt a bit." For me there was a reason to cry. And it did hurt! Rapport was not her strength, I'm afraid. In contrast, I've heard many nurses and pediatricians say to children, "I see your tears. This might hurt a bit. You'll feel a pinch but it will be quick and over." (This is a good start, but we can do even better, hypnotically speaking, as discussed in Chapter 8.)

Building Rapport With Pacing and Leading

Pacing	Leading
You look angry (worried, sad, uncomfortable) . . .	I wonder what we'll do about that. I wonder what might help.
Often the first few minutes plod along . . .	But let's see if the pace picks up!
Meeting someone for the first time can feel weird . . .	And then the next time we meet, it's not the first time. Think about that!
You probably don't know how this is going to go exactly . . .	And then when we're done, you'll know a lot more.

As Teleska and Sugarman (2013) explain, rapport is more than being caring and empathic. It requires seeing the many parts of the child and connecting to what is truly there, while avoiding the mistake of minimizing or denying the problem.

It's also interesting to switch the sequence a bit, and think about how being hypnotic builds rapport with children. Yapko described being hypnotic as being "so attuned and connected to the client that you are difficult to ignore and take lightly because what you're doing and what you're offering is so relevant and absorbing" (2012, p. 390). A child sitting in front of me, nervous about our first meeting or angry to be brought to see yet another professional, usually sits up and takes notice when I utter the words, "You know, I have a story about another girl like you who was here just this morning. . . . I'll tell you about her in a moment." A teenager pays close attention when I say deliberately, "Now let me repeat back to you what *you want* from these sessions. Listen *carefully and slowly*, because I want to make sure I've got it right." Even simply saying, "I am really focusing on what you're telling me" makes an impact.

I said earlier that separating out the interwoven components of the first encounter is tricky, and this is exactly what I mean. By being hypnotically attuned and absorbing, I'm building rapport and thus opening the door to immediate and future suggestions (Erickson & Rossi, 1979; Yapko, 2012). When I build rapport, I'm creating an environment that focuses attention (both mine and the client's) and draws us into the work at hand. Let's now add another ingredient of this first encounter: the observation of family patterns.

OBSERVATION OF CHILD AND FAMILY PATTERNS

Imagine for a moment two dogs or cats meeting for the first time. They spot each other and freeze, then begin to move slowly and deliberately. Their eyes adjust, ears and tails move, fur bristles. Vocalizations are deliberate and often unique. All parts of them join to communicate messages about status, threat, and territory. Who are you? What is your intent? What's your next move? They take their time deciphering the encounter, sizing each other up. It may only last a few seconds, but time seems suspended while much is shared.

Now imagine sitting next to a stranger on a plane, meeting a new colleague, or watching a toddler navigate a staircase. Where does your focus land? What absorbs your attention? What conclusions do you make? How do you determine what to do next? You base your responses on what you observe, what you deem significant, and how you then choose to react.

Creatures that interact with other creatures, from dachshunds to dentists to detectives, are well served by honing their observational skills. Clinicians using hypnosis with children should make this a priority. As Erickson and Rossi explained in the first chapter of *Hypnotherapy*, "new observational skills are the first stage in the training of the hypnotherapist" (1979, p. 15). They instructed the student of hypnosis to practice observing the following: role relations, how people behave within their frames of reference, the occurrence of everyday trance states, and response attentiveness. They described response attentiveness as a moment of openness to a suggestion or new frame of reference, a moment of openness when a person is "engaged in an inner search" (p. 17).

What do I mean when I talk about observing a family's frame of reference? Simply, it means noticing and gathering information about how the child (and family) understand and categorize the problem, and more generally how they move through life. How people react, interpret, or make conclusions about the events of their lives has been shown to greatly influence mental health and functioning. It is a predictor of depression, anxiety, physical health, and, on the brighter side, happiness, success, and healing (Beck, 1976; Beck, Rush, Shaw, & Emery, 1979; Yapko, 1992, 2001; Seligman, 1989, 1990, 1995, 2011). Paying attention to cognitive biases and attributional styles (for example, the depression-predicting stable-global-permanent triad) can influence the way that people make decisions, interact with others, recover from setbacks, and evaluate risk, just to name a few (Beck et al., 1979; Seligman, 1989; Kaslow, Stark, Printz, Livingston, & Shung, 1992).

The reality is that many of us, out of habit, busyness, or even years of experience and confidence, fall into the habit of not noticing.

Following well-worn pathways helps us to be efficient and streamlined. I needn't notice all the houses on my street as I drive to the bank, thereby freeing my brain to think of other things. I don't have to consider the exact words as I leave a "checking in" message on my sister's voice mail because we usually leave the same few sentences. With clients we may develop a familiar patter to greet them when they arrive at our office. While routine has its place, my goal is to push you out of your routine in the name of utilization and creativity (Haley, 1973). The more you observe and identify a family's frame of reference, the more targeted your hypnotic interventions and the better your therapy (Yapko, 2001).

As tempting as it is to say, "Observe everything!" it's not particularly instructive. Therefore, in this next section I describe two initial areas to focus upon when you meet a child and family, namely the occurrence of spontaneous trances and the use of imagination in families. In Chapter 4 I discuss in detail how to expand and use these observations as you identify common frames of reference and determine the targets of your interventions.

NOTICING NATURALLY OCCURRING TRANCE

As I began to learn about and experience the effectiveness of hypnosis, I wanted to use it as often as I could. What a versatile tool! My mind was filled with ideas about the possible applications in my clinical work. When I became a mom, it was even more interesting to use what I knew about hypnosis in the day-to-day parenting of my two boys. I could get them to listen, to cooperate, to settle down or go to sleep by grabbing hold of those naturally occurring trance states or everyday trances, as Milton Erickson called them. Rarely did I do a formal induction with my boys; I just waited for the right moment and planted seeds or suggestions.

I learned to notice and grab onto an emotional moment, a blank stare, or a heightened state of focus. Dropping my voice and launching into a story about the high price of stubbornness worked wonders when we needed to get out of the house on time or buckle up the car seat. (A stubborn little frog refused to listen to his mother's instruction to sit on the lily pad in their pond, and sadly missed the parade of fish, dragonflies, and marching waterbugs that went by. . . .) Talking slowly about how muscles and bones and eyelids and ears all know how to fall asleep when we send the "busy brain train" off on an adventure seemed like magic. Of course it wasn't magic; I was jumping at the opportunity to make suggestions during moments of spontaneous trance. (There are, and continue to be, many missed opportunities as well, I assure you.)

In 1966, Maria Montessori wrote about the experience of creating a trancelike silence in a classroom of young children:

> One day I entered the classroom holding in my arms a four-month-old baby girl that I had taken from her mother in the courtyard. The infant was tightly wrapped in swaddling bands as was the custom among the people of this neighborhood. Her face was full and rosy. She was so still that her silence impressed me greatly and I wanted the children to share my feelings. "She is not making a sound," I told them. And jokingly I added, "None of you could do so well." To my great surprise I saw that the children were looking at me with an extraordinary intensity. They seemed to be hanging on my lips and to be feeling keenly what I was saying. "Notice," I continued, "how soft her breath is. None of you could breathe as silently as she." Surprised and motionless, the children began to hold their breaths. At that moment there was an impressive silence. The tick-tock of the clock, which was not usually heard, began to become audible. It seemed as if the little girl had brought an atmosphere of silence into the room which is never found in daily life. (pp. 123–124)

This lovely story describes a naturally occurring trance when the children became spontaneously focused on the baby's quiet breath and then responded to their teacher's quiet suggestions.

Your first interactions with children and parents are ripe with opportunities to capitalize on these spontaneous trances. When parents and children first arrive for treatment, they may be experiencing a variety of emotional and cognitive states that enhance their openness to suggestion (Kuttner, 1988; Olness & Kohen, 1996; Kohen & Olness, 2011; Sugarman, 1996). A child who is anxious, curious, scared, or even excited is likely in a focused or attentive state, concentrating, watching, and absorbed in what's going to happen next. Picture the face of a child watching a juggler or waiting for the distant drummers in a parade to round the corner into sight. The gaze is fixed, muscles still, ears and eyes poised and ready. Berberich describes the naturally occurring trance of a child during a medical examination: "the cessation of activities, a captured gaze, slack facial features, and frozen posture" (2007, p. 124).

These receptive states have great value. Your words and actions can suggest comfort ("Find your spot on my comfortable couch"), make predictions ("I think this will be interesting"), promote action ("I'm ready to get going. How about you?"), or even confuse ("I wonder if this will be a long appointment that goes by quickly or a short appointment that goes by longly"). Your actions—taking a slow breath, holding eye contact and smiling, sitting silently for an extra moment, changing your seat unexpectedly—are examples of ways to focus attention and make subtle suggestions about what's to come. Such a trance moment may also cue you to be silent or gently "facilitate the inner search" (Erickson & Rossi, 1979) with a reinforcing statement like, "I see you're thinking" or "Imagine that."

As you read, allow your imagination to buzz with thoughts and examples of your own. What have you noticed in your recent sessions? What have you done, said, or modeled to take advantage of these moments of receptivity? Improving your ability to use these moments—and then determine what to say and what to do as you move forward—is what this book is all about.

What might you suggest if a child:

- Hides behind his parents when you greet them?
  I see you're taking your time before you let me see you. That's smart. Do you use your eyes to learn things? I know lots of animals that do that. . . . They watch and listen. . . . That can be very wise. . . .

- Stares at his feet and says nothing when you ask a question?
  You can take your time answering . . . or maybe you've already answered in your mind. . . . Just because you're quiet on the outside doesn't mean you're quiet on the inside. . . . You'll let me know when you're ready to answer on the outside, won't you? Are you thinking on the inside?

- Begins to tear up as you start the conversation?
  I see your tears, and tears are fine here. Tears can mean so many things. Maybe you know what your tears mean. Are there some feelings with the tears? Another girl told me she wished her tears could talk, and I told her that would be cool, but maybe she'd have to talk for her tears, and that made her smile a little. . . .

- Happily bounces around the room, looking in drawers?
  I wonder who is more curious, me or you? Can I learn some things about you while you learn some things about me and my office?

- Asks repeatedly what time she gets to leave?
  Are you thinking about what you get to do when you leave here? Can you tell me? We'll be done at 1:30. I have to be done then, too, so we can both pay a little bit of attention to the clock right there and also pay attention to each other so we can get our work done in time. I love having something to look forward to. . . .

Let me remind you that while these first chapters attune you to the building of the hypnotic atmosphere in your initial contacts, all of what I've described thus far will continue to be a part of your thinking and planning in every subsequent meeting with a child and her family.

IMAGINATION IN THE FAMILY

This entire book centers on the use of imagination, both yours and of the families you meet. Because you'll be inviting a family into the world of imagining, it is critical to observe how a child and family already engage these parts of themselves, both in the context of problem solving—or problem generating—and in their normal, day-to-day lives. As discussed in Chapter 2, your knowledge of child and adolescent development is an important first guide in understanding how children of certain ages and stages use imagination, metaphor, and fantasy. Add to this your observations of a child and parents' actual relationship and use of imagination to best determine how you can use this powerful resource. The family's use of imagination may enhance a child's ability to use hypnosis, but can also create some interesting dynamics between parent and child (LeBaron, 1983).

Questions to ask yourself as you assess the family's use of imagination:

- How does this family talk about the problem?
- Is their language concrete or more abstract?
- Do they use metaphors and similes to describe the symptoms or other aspects of their family life?
- Does the family engage in such activities as storytelling, role-playing, and imaginative play?
- Do they use stories as examples when talking about their problem?
- How detailed are their descriptions?
- Do they use their imagination in a negative or positive way?
- Do they have a sense of humor?

Sample questions to ask the child and family about the problem that will reveal information about their use of imagination:

- How big is this problem right now?
- If you could do anything, how would you make this problem go away?
- How will things be different when this problem isn't in charge?
- If this problem could talk, what would it say to me?
- Imagine yourself in a battle with this problem, and you can be anything in the world and the problem can be anything in the world. What would you both be? Tell me about the battle.
- Can you feel the problem in your body? Where does it live? What does it feel like?
- If you were an animal, what kind of animal would you be? What if the problem were an animal? What would it be?

My goal is to use the power of imagination to help discover solutions, but not in a general way that makes generic assumptions. (Try telling a child to imagine walking on a beach when she's never been to a beach or is afraid of sharks.) Asking questions like those listed above helps gauge the child's ability to think creatively about the issue and allows you to tailor your suggestions. Listen for interests, language, and level of creativity. Your most effective metaphors and images will come from the child's perceptions and language, not yours.

I remember asking a child what animal he would like to be, and how he imagined his problem. He said he wanted to be a bald eagle. He imagined his problem as a fish, and he would swoop down, grab it with his claws, and rip it apart with his beak. His most relaxing place, he said, was in the top of a tree in his backyard. "This is where I would sit and rip apart my fish," he said. Never in a million years would I have conjured up that image.

Be aware that not all children have great imaginations, as many want to presume. Some children are concrete in their thinking and thus struggle with metaphors and stories. I once asked an 8-year-old the "if you were an animal" question above, knowing that 8-year-olds are often capable of thinking in this metaphorical way. He looked at me with some confusion and answered, "But I'm not an animal. I'm a boy. I'm Dennis. Do you know how to help boys?" Another teen I worked with had a family who valued concrete information and evidence, and found it silly to imagine the stomach pain as anything other than pain in his stomach.

Also be aware that vivid imaginations are not always helpful. Some children have imaginations that pull them deeper into the problem, rather than out. LeBaron (1983) describes the use of hypnotic interventions with high-fantasy children as potentially upsetting when dealing with illness or pain, because these children create negative imagery focused on pain or death. A 6-year-old girl I treated used her imagination to repeatedly imagine her own kidnapping in such detail that she would scream and tremble at bedtime every night, often until she vomited. Anxious children and anxious parents commonly imagine worst-case scenarios and catastrophic outcomes; therefore imagination enhancement will be productive only if it heads in the right direction.

Your awareness of a child's imaginative style increases your effectiveness. If a child has a concrete style of thinking or is too young to pull meaning from a story and relate it to his own problem, you may need to explain the reason for your story and help him make the connection (Yapko, 2012). Your goal might then be to model how stepping into his imagination can flexibly aid with a solution. For a child whose symptom is a direct result of a too-vivid imagination, you may choose to teach distance from this powerful part of her when needed. How to move away from the scary images—and how to differentiate between helpful creativity and scary wanderings—would be an important skill to develop. I'll continue to talk ever more specifically about how to customize your client's imagination for specific circumstances.

SUGGESTIVE INTERVIEWING:
USING WORDS THAT MATTER

My first job after graduate school was on an acute inpatient psychiatric unit in a teaching hospital. In this medical setting, I learned a great deal about assessment. My job as the novice social worker was to do a biopsychosocial interview on each new patient and write up a thorough intake for the chart. I gathered important information for the team, but as I think back on it now, I did nothing intentional during that interaction to shift the patient's perspective or orient him toward a positive outcome. The questions I asked had likely been answered many times before: family history, job, current living situation, past treatment experiences.

Maybe these interactions were helpful in some way because I listened empathically or did my best to be energetic and kind. Nonetheless, I was completely unaware of the potential of these interviews. My unidirectional and formulaic approach yielded cursory data, at best (Berberich, 2011).

My definition of an assessment was too limited. I asked questions and gathered lots of data, but I wasn't harnessing the potential of these conversations. I became a better clinician when, because of my training in hypnosis and strategic therapy, my own frame shifted. I began to tune into the potential power of initial meetings, to recognize that no encounter is unidirectional and that I could begin to intervene immediately. As Zeig wrote, "Assessment is intervention. . . . Assessment has an impact. . . . One needs a general sense of where one is directing the treatment but clinicians don't need to have massive amounts of specific data to begin to intervene. . . . Early intervention communicates to the patient that psychotherapy is about change and doing things differently more than it is about understanding" (2006, p. 57).

It is obviously important to gather information about a child in order to best treat him. As I explained above, immediately noticing how a family describes and understands the issue is hugely valuable. But the point here is that when you are in front of a child for the first time—a child who is likely in an enhanced state of focus and suggestibility—your interactions should be directed toward potential and change, or what Erickson and Rossi described as "depotentiating a patient's learned limitations" (1979, p. 6). Even before you fully know the details, content, or framework of a problem, your questions, your comments, and the way in which you go about learning a child's story are the start of your treatment, a nod toward the future. Your goal is to engage a family and use language that will, for example:

- Create expectancy and hopefulness
- Employ the imagination and a spirit of play
- Suggest malleability and flexibility as a new frame
- Shift the child and family toward the future
- Activate existing or past resources
- Spark curiosity and predict uncertainty

Can you think of a presenting problem that wouldn't benefit from the introduction of such concepts? Think for a moment about either a significant or run-of-the-mill problem, and the potential impact of approaching the problem with this frame of mind. Suppose, for example, you take your new puppy to an obedience class. The puppy trainer's opening speech is engaging. Imagine he helps you envision the end result of your training, makes you curious about what you and your puppy are going to learn, and exudes hopefulness about your success in the class. You'd listen for the information, ready to follow the instructions, wouldn't you?

I frequently do small, intensive workshops for parents who are dealing with anxiety in their families, six hours over two nights. The parents arrive concerned, tired, and often frustrated, but also hopeful and eager to learn. As I begin, during those first few minutes, I am purposefully hypnotic. It goes like this:

Welcome. . . . I've chatted with many of you already . . . and I know how focused you are on helping your child and your family . . . so you've made it here tonight. . . . I know how much effort and planning that takes. . . . Take a breath! . . . Settle in and get ready to learn and absorb. . . . I'm wondering how many of you know how worry works. . . . Have you had someone walk through the steps of how it operates? . . . A few of you. . . . The truth is this . . . it's not complicated . . . and as big and overwhelming as it feels right now . . . in your house . . . in your family . . . by the end of these two nights you will understand how it works and what to do. . . . I have slides . . . a whiteboard. . . . I brought chocolate. . . . You'll do some homework assignments. . . . I know you've been stuck . . . but I have information and you have skills. . . . Be prepared to hear some things I'm guessing will be different from what you've been taught before. . . . I predict . . . looking ahead . . . by the end of our time together . . . you'll be better equipped. . . . So let's dive in. . . .

This section focuses on asking questions and using language in the initial interview that tie together what I've described above: words that build rapport, make the most of naturally occurring trance, promote flexibility, and begin to reveal the target for your interventions (which I cover in detail in Chapter 4). When we aim to alleviate a child's distress as quickly as possible, we're off to a quicker start by recognizing and using these hypnotic interactions from the first meeting. As Kohen and Olness wrote, "Consider viewing history taking as rapport building, that is future (not just past) oriented, strength based, change based (vs. stuck), and positively expectant" (2011, p. 109).

If you are in the early stages of using hypnosis with children—or even if you've been working hypnotically for decades—this may sound ambitious (or overwhelming). My advice as you build your skills is this: focus on one or two aspects of the initial interview at a time. Set a goal for yourself: "I will focus on noticing a naturally occurring trance state" or "I will ask questions that are future oriented." I learned this type of self-training from Dr. Jeff Zeig (personal communication, 2007), who writes of Erickson's model of lifelong self-development and who teaches this model in his own trainings and classes. And in a broader sense, this is how most everyone learns to improve a particular craft, be it playing a piano, doing mathematics, or playing football. Focus on one or two skills at a time until they become part of your muscle memory or thinking repertoire, then move on to the next.

The bottom line: your precise use of suggestive language as you ask questions, make observations, and promote new (and improved) frameworks will improve your interventions. My children's magical kindergarten teacher, Mary (gifted in the use of all of the above) reminded and modeled for parents that we must always speak impeccably when speaking with children. The following sections address this use of language in more detail.

Expectancy and Hopefulness

Expectations are powerful. Erickson and Rossi (1979, p. 3) describe expectancy as "a singularly important aspect" in creating the "optimal attitude" as one prepares to work with a client hypnotically. As I said earlier, the impact of negative and positive expectations on health and healing, mood, and even sports performance is well-documented (Nolen-Hoeksema, Girgus, & Seligman, 1992; Seligman, Nolen-Hoeksema, Thorton, & Thornton, 1990). Negative anticipation of bad things happening, or a stuck belief that bad situations never change, make up the core of anxiety and depression (Kaslow et al., 1992). Anxious children imagine the worst and thus work to avoid the discomfort of their well-rehearsed catastrophe, seeing themselves as unable to cope (Barlow, 2001). Depressed people expect situations or people or themselves to disappoint (for some, strengthened by their past experiences), and add salt to the wound with a dose of hopelessness about anything changing in the future (Beck, Rush, Shaw, & Emery, 1979; Abramson, Metalsky, & Alloy, 1989; Joiner, 2000).

Positive expectations can be just as influential. In David McRaney's (2011) book *You Are Not So Smart*, he recounts a study done with undergraduates in "wine school" who were told to describe in detail a cheap wine secretly placed in an expensive bottle. They loved it, calling it "complex and rounded." When they were given the same cheap wine in a cheap bottle, they were not at all impressed.

A study of consumer packaging found that buyers had more positive reactions to a product's packaging when it included a picture of the product itself (Underwood & Klein, 2002). A study looking at recovery from neck pain found a strong relationship between a patient's positive expectation of complete pain relief and the success of physical therapy (Bishop, Mintken, Bialosky, & Cleland, 2013).

In his 2009 book *The Emperor's New Drugs: Exploding the Antidepressant Myth*, Irving Kirsch, an expert on the placebo effect, described multiple studies illustrating how expectations influenced the outcomes of antidepressant drug trials, arthroscopic knee surgeries, asthma, and even reactions to poison ivy. His work with Steven Jay Lynn and others (Lynn & Kirsch, 2006; Kirsch et al., 2008; Kirsch, 1985, 1999, 2000, 2005b, 2005c) illuminates the power of response expectancies on both our psychological and physical states.

So what does this mean clinically? That the use of a formal versus informal hypnotic procedure with a child becomes ultimately less important than how you create the positive expectancy of what can and will happen (Lynn, 2007; Lynn & Kirsch, 2006; Lynn,

Neufeld, & Maré, 1993). Your primary focus must be on the fostering of a state of belief that maximizes the powerful impact of your words and interactions (Kirsch, 2000; Kirsch & Lynn, 1997).

Children and parents arrive with all sorts of expectations, both positive and negative: "Therapy is so stupid; no one can help me; she's going to make me talk about difficult stuff; talking doesn't help anything; this is going to hurt; I'm in trouble; this is boring" or "I've heard good things about Lynn Lyons; I get to miss school; I hope she knows what to do; my friend said she can help; she knows what she's doing." Both parents and children are waiting to see how their expectations line up with the reality of this first encounter. Your job is to use the language of positive expectancy and to convey to the family that you expect improvement and have the skills to help (Yapko, 2001, 2012).

Based on what you know and what you see, tailor your expressions of positive expectancy to the energy level and personality of the child in front of you. During these first moments, emotions and anticipation are often piqued. While some children are sitting wide eyed as if waiting for a birthday cake to come around the corner, other children are anticipating your introduction like the next crack of thunder during a storm. (Imagine these two faces for a few seconds, and picture the spontaneous trance. Recognize how hypnotic this moment can be.)

Pessimistic, resistant, and treatment-weary kids need a more measured approach. They are skeptical that you can help. They are looking for a reason to categorize you as anything from clueless to naive about the depth of their issues. ("She's not gonna want to hear about how bad I feel" or "She's way too positive. She's not like me. She doesn't understand what this is like.") If your enthusiasm and optimism come across as fake, overwhelming, or incongruous, they may think you are not seeing them as individuals, but offering your generic sales pitch.

Sixteen-year-old Meghan came to see me for severe stress-induced headaches. When I welcomed her into my office, she moved slowly and her eyes were almost closed. "I can see your discomfort. It's helpful for me to see that. When someone arrives with a headache, I get a clearer picture of what to do. We'll talk a bit, then I'll show you how this works." A few meetings later, when Meghan's headaches were on the decline, she shared, "When I met you, you didn't make huge promises. But you said you knew what to do. And you also knew I was really in pain."

In contrast, Maya, a 10-year-old with lots of worries, jumped up happily when I greeted her and her mom in the waiting room. She turned to her mom and practically cheered, "Here she is! Lynn Lyons!" My response was equally enthusiastic. "After talking to your mom and your teacher, I was expecting a friendly, smiling girl like you. I also hear you have a great imagination. I'm so excited to hear all about it." Maya responded with, "My teacher said she met you. She said you were funny and that you knew how to handle worries. Can you show me?" Her expectation was that we get right to work, so off we went to discover how she could fix her worry monster.

Talking About the Future

Asking questions that direct a family toward the future is inseparable from the creation of hope and positive expectancy; therefore "moving forward" suggestions and questions will increase the success of your interventions (Kessler & Miller, 1995). In a therapy setting, many children (especially teens) will come to you with the belief that treatment consists of talking about what has happened already. Many adults still have the antiquated perception that therapy consists of endlessly analyzing your mother and your childhood, dissecting and understanding the wounds of the past. Immediately establishing that you intend to look forward (where change can happen) is often a relief for children who would rather not endure another cataloguing of their failures—or more history taking.

I have an opening question that I ask almost every person who comes to see me, inspired by Insoo Kim Berg and Steve de Shazer's (1988) well-known miracle question:

> *Imagine that it's six months or even a year from now, and you're telling someone about this experience . . . these visits we will have together. And you say—when you're talking about this experience several months from now—"I went to see Lynn, and it was really successful/helpful because . . ." Can you finish that sentence for me?*

Not only does the answer clarify the hopes of the child or parent, but it reveals my orientation as well: the question pulls them into the future, presupposes success (in a relatively short period of time), and engages the imagination. The answer may be global ("I want to feel better") or completely different than what Mom told me on the phone. And more than a few kids have said, "It will be successful because I don't have to come here anymore." Every response helps me identify the expectations and ask follow-up questions that consistently focus on the desired goal.

"I want to feel better" leads to a more specific question: "So when I see you in 6 months or 3 weeks and you do feel better, what will you tell me then? What will be different?"

"My mom wants me to do better in school but I want to have fun with my friends" leads to a collaborative statement: "When the two of you figure this out together, I wonder what that will look like."

"I don't have to come here anymore" leads to rapport building: "That's my goal, too: to work myself out of a job. Let's get to work on making that happen."

Tolerating Uncertainty, Creating Flexibility

The questions above guide a child toward a different future, imagining how life can change compared to what she is experiencing now.

This new framework is critical to treat the many problems children present to us: depression, anxiety, chronic pain or illness, and grief and loss. These children must have hope that tomorrow can look and feel different than today. A child in the first months of his parents' contentious separation has difficulty conceiving of a time when he won't feel so sad and angry about the changes he must endure. Planting a suggestive seed that he has the capacity to adapt to the changes in his present and future life is a helpful message to drop during a bleak and uncertain time.

But telling a child that tomorrow will be better is not enough— and sometimes not accurate. The ability to accept and tolerate the uncertainty of the future is an important skill that helps children ultimately step into new situations, take on reasonable risks, establish social connections, and handle life's unexpected events. Depressed and anxious children in particular need this skill of tolerating uncertainty as a way out of their rigid and pessimistic frames (Seligman, 1995). Although it might sound contradictory to focus a child on what he wants in the future while also letting him know that the future is uncertain, this type of flexibility allows a child to move forward rather than avoid the uncertainty of new and unfamiliar experiences (Wilson & Lyons, 2013). In fact, you probably use this approach all the time. Think about a goal you set for yourself, and the flexibility required to make it happen.

Brendan came to see me when he was 9. His mom had recently told him that his family was moving to a nearby town. Even though he could certainly visit his friends, it meant starting another school, adapting to a new neighborhood, and playing on a different soccer team. Brendan was angry and worried. His mother repeatedly reassured him that he would make new friends, and that the new school was a better fit in a better neighborhood, but this only made him angrier. "She keeps telling me it will be great. How does she know?" My response surprised him. "She can't know, actually. She can hope, and guess, and plan. But she can't know. You can't either. Maybe we can make a list of what will help you at your new school—like some buddies to play with at recess and a way to still see your old buddies—and then come up with some ideas. But we can't know who will be your friends yet. How can we know? You do know that you're good at making friends, though, right?"

The language of flexibility and the ability to tolerate not knowing in this context say to a family, "You know what you want, and we can expect to get there, but we must also figure out the details along the way." When you use the language of flexibility, you model and foreshadow skills that children will need as they step into this arena of change, namely the ability to learn, shift, and adapt along the way. You're also letting the child know that you are not the expert on him or his problems. You have experience and knowledge, but you'll need his input and ideas.

Examples of such phrases (mine and others):

- "I wonder where you would rather be than here" (Sugarman & Wester, 2013, p. 9).
- To a child about to have surgery: "I answered by telling him with a smile that I didn't know how it was going to feel for HIM. I didn't know if it was going to feel like an ache, or an itch, or a sore muscle" (Lobe, 2013, p. 384).
- "I don't know how you'll do that" (Kohen & Murray, 2006, p. 209) or "I'm not sure how you will DO that" (p. 196).
- "I have some ideas, but I'm still learning about you. What else do you want me to know?"
- "I'm so interested to see what we'll discover together. Any guesses?"

Accessing Resources

When talking earlier about gathering history, I wrote that the extensive reporting of past failures (although illustrative of a family's framework) tends to set a not-so-helpful tone in an initial meeting.

Out of necessity you will hear some history about the problem with the child present, ideally from the child herself. But no child's history is all bad; therefore take advantage of this first meeting to introduce the value of both recognizing existing resources and viewing past experiences as learning opportunities that inform the future.

When human beings are struggling—and even when they're not—scanning for and recalling positives doesn't come easy or naturally. The negativity bias in our primitive brains is designed to ensure our survival (Baumeister, Bratslavsky, Finkenauer, & Vohs, 2001). As Rick Hanson described in his book *Hardwiring Happiness*, this bias creates "Velcro for bad experiences, but Teflon for good ones" (2013, p. 27). In my daily clinical work with anxious children, I see how they are amnesiac to past success while often catastrophically predicting future failure. If a problem has been long-standing, a child may be acutely aware of her inability to fix it, and wary of another conversation that suggests her stubbornness, resistance, or lack of motivation. Perhaps solutions have been offered, and adults have become frustrated by the behavior's apparent imperviousness to discipline or consequence. Thus the seed of possible, positive change must be planted early—and it may meet some resistance.

In such circumstances, joining a child by acknowledging the reality of the problem but then (gently) predicting the discovery or creation of positive resources builds further rapport and creates positive momentum. This is similar to the pacing and leading discussed earlier. Your goal is to convey the idea, "This problem has a solution and we're about to begin an interesting search." Language infused with curiosity and even uncertainty, as described in the previous section, can work well: "I don't know exactly what we'll find or what's needed, but let's search together."

Ten-year-old Jenna was having trouble with her peers on the playground, often pushing them to the ground and yelling at them. Jenna's behavior was consistently triggered by being left out, but her reaction was only creating the result she most feared: more rejection. Jenna understood this when discussing the events afterward, but in the moment couldn't stop this ingrained behavior. When I met Jenna, I could have said, "I know you're a nice girl deep inside, and you don't want to hurt your classmates." But this would have only confirmed to Jenna (who was very ashamed of her behavior) that I, like the other adults, didn't understand the power of her feelings and thought that she could just stop if she wanted to enough. The message, "You're nice! Be nice!" gave her nothing but more shame and confusion. Instead, I said, "It sounds like you have a powerful part inside of you that gets very angry. It's not helping you make friends right now, so maybe we'll have to discover how to handle that part when it wants to be in charge. Maybe there's something else inside you that will help with that." This tells Jenna that we're about to go on a search. In fact, in that moment, the search has already begun.

Other examples of phrases or questions that suggest the discovery, retrieval, or creation of positive resources include:

- I'm not sure exactly what we're going to do yet, but after talking to you for a bit, I'm excited to look for some solutions.
- What are you good at? How did you get good at it? Is there anything from there that we can use to help us over here?
- Is there anything else I should know about you . . . something that will help us find a solution to this?
- I'm curious about times when this problem didn't show up. I wonder how that happened.
- What's already inside you that will help?
- When something changes, what will change?
- Let's imagine that there is a big, beautiful store . . . and it's called the Solution Store, and in this store you'll find the solution to this problem of [state child's problem]. Just imagine for a moment that you're walking through the aisles of the store. Where would we find the solution? Any idea what it would be?

If a child answers, "I don't know" to some of these questions, I sometimes shrug and reply, "I don't know either. Not yet, anyway. I wonder if we can imagine or guess, and then we can not know together for a time while we find out" (adapted from Teleska & Sugarman, 2013).

There are also circumstances when confidence in finding a solution needs to be more directly conveyed. Even though we hope the child will ultimately access his own internal resources, a direct and confident suggestion to a family in distress can work wonders. For example, 9-year-old Eli arrived with his worried mother for help with chronic vomiting. Mom recounted their experiences thus far: after an extensive medical examination found no organic etiology, the pediatrician announced to both of them, "You're a mystery to me, Eli. I have no idea what's going on with you." Within a few minutes, I actually did know what was going on with Eli (from an anxiety perspective it was clear) and chose to let them both know that I was familiar with this problem and had some strategies to teach them. "Eli, I know this problem well. You can learn how to take charge," I told him, "and with your great imagination and what I know about how worry works, we're going to take care of this together."

You have now learned to:

- Build rapport
- Begin your observation of spontaneous trance and imagination
- Use suggestive language that begins movement toward change
- Be hypnotic from the start and utilize what the child offers

The goal of this chapter is to help you appreciate and harness the power of your initial contact. We talked about the key steps of both absorbing information and priming the child and family for change. So much is gained by using the heightened emotional state and openness of these first moments.

CASE EXAMPLES: THE INITIAL GREETING
WITH PETER AND ALEXIS

The following contrasting case examples of Peter and Alexis—different scenarios with initially different expectations and levels of clarity—illustrate how to use and embrace hypnotic opportunities in the first moments of the encounter. In each case, I build rapport by acknowledging the issue, dealing with the expectations (positive and negative) that the family brings to the appointment, and by being attuned to the child's words and emotions.

Peter's mother calls to schedule an appointment because Peter, a 15-year-old high school student, has been having panic attacks before tests at school. Mom previously suggested therapy to help, but he refused because "therapy is stupid and embarrassing." Peter then heard about hypnosis from a friend who said it could help him do better on tests. Peter urged his mother to call for an appointment, because hypnosis is "cool," unlike therapy.

Seven-year-old Alexis has been having difficulty falling asleep at night. Her parents have tried everything they can think of, but despite their efforts, she is routinely awake until 11:00 P.M. The pediatrician recommended they get some therapy for Alexis, and Mom calls for an appointment, hoping that I can teach Alexis some "better strategies to fall asleep" and address some of Alexis's other "behavior issues." The sleep issue, says Mom, "might just be the tip of the iceberg."

After the initial conversations with each mother, I contemplate how I will use hypnosis as a part of my treatment plan, and how I will approach this in the first session. These cases are so different from each other. Peter wants hypnosis. I can assume that he expects some ritual and formality that fit his image of the hypnotic experience. Peter sees hypnosis as distinct from other treatments, and certainly distinct from therapy. He knows what he wants: to manage the panic and do better on tests. Because of his age, he'll probably want to meet alone. And I must be careful to avoid the term *therapy*.

On the other hand, I don't know what Alexis expects or wants. Does she want to come for help? Does she even see a problem? I anticipate her parents will be present for at least part of the session. I know there's a sleep problem, but I'm in the dark about the other behavioral issues. Mom's language indicates that she's feeling a bit overwhelmed by her daughter, and that many attempts at a solution have failed. They did not seek me out, as far as I know, for hypnosis. What are their perceptions of hypnosis? What are they expecting?

When Peter arrives with his mother, I greet them in the waiting room and we exchange introductions. As we chat, I hand Peter the paperwork on a clipboard, a brief intake form to read and complete with the instruction, "Mom can help out if needed, and then you both must sign the bottom." He completes it with a few questions for Mom, and I ask Peter if he'd like Mom to join us to start, or if Mom has any questions for me. Mom holds up her hand like a traffic cop, smiles, and shakes her head. "He's all set," she says. "Should I wait here or come back?" Peter tells her she can go, but I tell her she can wait in the waiting room or go, but please return 60 minutes into our 90-minute session.

In my office I ask Peter my opening question: "In 6 months someone asks you about this experience, and you say, 'It was successful because . . .' How would you complete that statement?" Peter answers, "The panic stopped getting in the way of tests. I'm getting higher grades."

He is clear about the problem and his goal. He is concrete in his framing of the problem, and does not bring up any other times when the panic shows up, although there may be other contexts that he's not disclosing. He's a bit rigid in his focus and expectations, but not controlling. His mother is supportive of Peter's plan and willing to let

him handle it. I don't know yet how Peter has handled other problems in the past, but he is active in his approach to managing this,
and is focusing on success in his future.

"That's clear. Let's get to work," I say to Peter. "Ready to try something new? Ready for some hypnosis?"

Rapport Building	Message/Suggestion
Peter fills out the paperwork.	You are responsible and mature.
Peter decides if Mom stays or goes.	You are autonomous. This is your time.
"In six months, someone asks you . . ."	Future orientation.
"Let's get to work."	You are here to do something. You are looking for results. We're going to be efficient.
"Ready to try something new? Ready for some hypnosis?"	A direct invitation. A new (and flexible) approach. I understand what you want. The process begins now.

Alexis also has a concrete problem—being unable to fall
asleep—but there are indications throughout that there's more going
on. Mom is unsure about what to do, and the problem is defined as
"the tip of the iceberg." Icebergs are huge and their dangerous bulk
hides under water.

When I go to greet Alexis and her parents in the waiting
room, Alexis is standing with her arms crossed, looking at the
floor. She does not respond verbally to my hello, but looks up
quickly and then back down. "Alexis is not happy about being
here," Mom says.

"Yes, I see that. Some kids are curious, some kids are mad, some kids are actually excited, and some are nervous. Lots of kids are all of the above. It's okay. You don't know me and I don't know you, and you're supposed to talk about stuff, so it can feel weird at first. Normal. Some kids even have some tears. Trying not to cry can be very exhausting, though."

We decide that Alexis and her parents will come in together to start, but we might ask someone to leave later if we choose. Alexis says nothing as we make this decision and remains quiet and withdrawn.

Mom has been active, it appears, in her attempts to solve the sleep problem, but also talks about how the issues with Alexis are more pervasive. "I'm not sure" is a common answer and Mom says she is worried and overwhelmed at times. Alexis sits close to her mom, hiding her face much of the time in Mom's arm. She says very little. Based on her age, I'm not yet sure if she's usually this dependent upon her parents or if her behavior is the result of being in my office. She is unsure and not overtly willing—at this point—to participate in this process of change.

I say to everyone, "I just don't know exactly how it will go yet." Then to Alexis, "Do you have any pets?"

A dog and a cat, she answers. I ask her about them and she fills me in on their names, breeds, and personalities. "I have two cats," I tell her. "They like to sit on top of people's cars. You might see them when you leave. They're too naughty to come into the office. They scratch my chairs. Other than that they're friendly."

I tell her about a boy who brings his dog to our appointments and another girl who brought her bird in its cage one time.

"You let kids bring their pets?"

"When it helps," I answer. "Different things help different kids. And it's fun for me to see animals, too." (Had Alexis told me she did not have any pets, I might have engaged her, for example, in a conversation about cats and their curiosity, and that while I welcome curiosity in my office, cats also love to scratch furniture, and therefore mine have to stay outside.)

Rapport Building	Message/Suggestion
"Lots of kids are all of the above. It's okay."	You can feel all sorts of emotions. That's okay with me. It's normal.
"Trying not to cry can be very exhausting, though."	Everyone is trying to hold it together and that's tiring. There's a sleep issue; therefore "exhausting" is a word this family can relate to.
"I just don't know exactly how it will go yet."	We're in the same boat. We can be flexible. We're not supposed to know everything.
"Do you have any pets?"	We can talk about regular things, too. A little surprise question to shift.
"You might see them when you leave."	This will be over. Let's imagine the future for a minute. (And the story engages imagination.)
"They're too naughty to come into my office."	You can feel all sorts of things, but there are some behavioral expectations while here.
"It's fun for me to see animals, too."	We can be playful while we deal with these problems.

In both cases, building rapport is not (and cannot be) separate from careful use of language and word choice. Suggestions about flexibility, normalizing the process of working on a problem, supporting the autonomy of a child, and acknowledging the anxiety (or exhaustion, frustration, embarrassment) of children and parents are all done informally and immediately.

Treating Peter like a young adult with a clear goal in mind supports his active approach to addressing his panic. Because avoidance and passivity are often the strategies that anxious kids (and adults) adopt, I want to support an active framework directly. Alexis is much younger and the family is more overtly overwhelmed and emotional about the problem. I'm not sure what's going on (other than the sleep issue); therefore, normalizing the uncertain feelings and changing the family's tense emotional tone (with a little surprise question) in this first visit is essential. Mom referenced other behavioral problems in the phone call, which cues me to put some structure around behavior in the office.

AND FINALLY . . .

Michele Ritterman (1983) poetically described the interplay of rapport, observation, and language as a key to being welcomed rapidly into a family system, so that seeding for change can begin immediately. By communicating to the family her recognition of how each member understands the problem, she connects to the family; by being careful to acknowledge but not fall into the rigid, symptomatic patterns of the family, she creates a hypnotic atmosphere that suggests a new way of interacting. Her goal from the outset is "to ensure a minimum of rigid response" from the family. "The initial uncertainty about the therapist's role," she wrote, "is best transformed into excitement, enthusiasm, curiosity, and, when appropriate, anticipation into a major life-transforming event" (pp. 47–48).

Armed with information and inspiration, we're ready to move

forward. Chapter 4 delves deeper into the creation of your tailored hypnotic interventions. Building upon what you've observed and the seeds you've planted, you now must decide what to say and do in a hypnosis session. We'll talk in detail about identifying and prioritizing your therapeutic targets, and the five recurrent frames that will help to structure your sessions.

CHAPTER *4*

Know Where You're Headed

Targets and Frames

Seventeen-year-old Jane sits crying on the couch in front of me, tired from the recent battles of her parents' contentious divorce and worried about her own college plans. "I'm so sick of hearing my parents' negative voices in my head. I don't want to take those voices to college with me. I'm so different from them. I just don't see life through their miserable eyes."

Fourteen-year-old Anne has a severe phobia of vomiting. Since elementary school, her friends and family—knowing of this fear—have worked to protect her from any mention of vomit or exposure to it. With her permission and urging over the years, her team is vigilant. Anne has made some progress, but still views herself as fragile and demands that her friends and family monitor the environment for possible triggers.

Jane and Anne have very different approaches to their challenges. While Jane is clear about her desire to distance herself from negative family patterns as she heads off to college, Anne isn't yet ready to step away from her fearful—albeit safer—self-view. If your job is to help both girls move forward, where do you begin? What do you teach? And how? In this chapter I'll talk about how to take what a child and her parents offer about the presenting problem, and then figure out what to do with that information.

SHIFTING THE FRAMES

Decades of cognitive-based research show us that addressing how people react, interpret, or make conclusions about the events of their lives greatly influences their mental and physical health. With confidence we can predict that certain negative ways of thinking—notably the attributional styles of being internal ("It's my fault"), global ("Everything is lousy"), and stable ("It's not going to change")—create and maintain depression in both adults and children (Seligman, 1989; Nolen-Hoeksema et al., 1992). Overgeneralization and catastrophic thinking create anxiety in children (Weems, Berman, Silverman, & Saavedra, 2001; Weems, Costa, Watts, Taylor, & Cannon, 2007) and Beck's (1976) negative cognitive triad of feeling badly about oneself, the world, and the future has been shown to manifest as both anxiety and depression in children (Kaslow et al., 1992).

On the flip side, positive psychology research shows us how certain perceptions and interpretations create resilience. Seligman (1995, 2011) was able to identify the ways in which optimistic children interpret good and bad events differently than pessimistic children, how parents impact these explanatory styles, and thus how to "immunize" kids with this optimistic framework. Researchers have found that the number of stressful events one experiences does not consistently predict anxiety, physical symptoms, or other mental health issues. Much more important to well-being is how we interpret those events and whether or not we perceive the related stress as negative or positive (Rapee, Litwin, & Barlow, 1990; Wilson et al., 2011).

I suggested in Chapter 3 that developing the skill of recognizing a child's existing frames of reference become a priority. Getting a picture of how a child views herself, the issues that brought her to you, and her world in general enables you together to recognize where she gets stuck, create a different perspective, and capitalize on any positive frames that already exist (Erickson & Rossi, 1979). The goal of this chapter is to help you do just that, using hypnotic techniques and language as your primary method of delivery. Quite simply, I want you to be able to hear where a child is stuck, determine where he needs to go instead, and offer an alternative framework (of thinking, perceiving, acting) that shows him the way. As Yapko wrote, "The times when hypnosis in particular, and therapy in general works best are when there is a target to be hit and a well-defined means for doing so" (2001, p. 28).

In order to determine the best course of your interventions, you must first seek to better understand:

1. How this problem "lives" with a child and a family, and how you are going to offer a different (more helpful) "living arrangement" or a better range of choices (Zeig, 1988, 2006).
2. What resources and strategies already exist within the family and child, and what needs to be developed (Yapko, 2001, 2012).
3. How to introduce, teach, or amplify these resources during your treatment interactions (Erickson & Rossi, 1979; Yapko, 2001).

Once you recognize the frame(s) of the problem, your next job is to offer a new way of reacting, which means focusing your effective hypnotic interventions on the goal of shaking up the stuck patterns that are maintaining the problem (Zeig, 2006; Yapko, 2001). You may do this by utilizing existing resources and helping the client to activate them in a productive way, or, as Zeig states, "providing new information that the [family] may not have had at [their] disposal"

(2006, p. 93). This alternative frame may, for example, amplify Jane's desire to be more optimistic than her parents or help Anne actively take steps away from her fragile and dependent view of herself. By injecting flexibility of perspective, you become, first and foremost, the ambassador for change and possibility.

Below are descriptions and examples of the three broad frameworks that I consistently introduce to children and their parents. These alternative frames are not new; they define the work of past luminaries and current experts in strategic, cognitive, and hypnotic approaches—teachers that I reference throughout this book. They are so often a focus of my interventions because they are brilliantly ubiquitous and applicable, and because many of the issues that children and families present to us can be attributed to absences or deficits in these areas, as you'll see in the upcoming chapters.

After each frame, I provide questions to ask yourself as you evaluate the presenting problems. Look and listen for beliefs, perceptions, and patterns of a child's experience, all of which will determine the focus of your interventions. You may hear, for example, rigidity as a family talks about the problem ("We have rules to follow, and we don't understand why he needs to do it his own way") or a paralysis that begs for some action ("I don't want to do anything . . . and there's nothing to do anyway. . . . What am I supposed to do? I'm just a kid!").

The Three Frames

- Experience is variable (vs. rigid and permanent)
- The value of parts (vs. global and overwhelming)
  - Sequencing
  - Compartmentalizing
  - Connection and disconnection, or signals and noise
- Action counts (vs. passive and avoidant)

Experience Is Variable

Ten-year-old Adam and his family were preparing for a trip to Florida, about a 3-hour plane ride from Boston. He wasn't sure he could do it. "I might freak out. What if we hit bumps?"

He had flown several times before and it was routinely a struggle for him emotionally. "And also," he said, "Evelyn [his sister] loves to fly. I don't get it. How can she love it? How can anyone love it?"

"Well, I have a few thoughts about that interesting question, if you'd like to listen," I said. "You can listen with eyes open or closed. Either way is fine with me. Just a matter of personal preference."

Adam sat back. His eyes open and closed periodically as I continued:

People's preferences are so curious. . . . Some people find scary movies entertaining, while other people are just scared and wonder who would choose to feel that way. . . . Some people love spicy food, but other people just feel the pain and miss the flavor . . . or some kids hate shrimp for years and then try it again and love it . . . or how about the people who love to get up early and go for a run, but their friends see that as torture and want to sit comfortably with a cup of coffee? When you're playing with your best friend, the time goes by so fast. . . . You can't believe it when your mom shows up to get you . . . but in math class, seconds feel like minutes, and minutes feel like hours. . . . How can those minutes be the same and feel so different? And when your sister flies . . . she thinks about where she's headed . . . or feels the waves of air . . . or gets to order a soda that's not allowed at home . . . so she feels free. . . . And it's the same movie or the same food, same morning, same minute, same plane . . . on the outside. . . . It just can be different on the inside. . . . You can experiment with that sometimes.

Amplifying the theme of variability of experience is helpful on so many levels that I recommend doing it early and often. Not only does it give the child permission to experience his time with you in many different ways, but lets him know that what he is thinking or feeling is both fine with you and perhaps capable of shifting. Does Adam have to love flying? No, but maybe he can shift the experience in a way that makes it manageable. Or maybe he'll have a different experience that will actually change his mind or allow him to look at the freedom of being on a plane (perhaps to have a special soda of his own). Who knows?

By the way, Adam wasn't seeing me because he had a fear of flying. He was having difficulty with peers at school because of his shyness. He had developed a habit of growling at kids that asked him to participate in any activity that he perceived as stupid. Getting him to take some risks socially and experiment with different activities was an important goal. He needed to work on more flexible responses to others, and the ability to accept others' ideas and perceptions, even when different from his own. I was always listening for opportunities to address his rigid framework, so I welcomed his worry about the plane trip and his frustration with Evelyn's point of view as another opportunity to guide this shift.

Introducing hypnotic phenomena in an interesting or fun way also creates a real-life, in-the-moment experience of variability. Having a child imagine and experience the sensation of her hand becoming heavier or lighter, or salivating as she imagines biting into a lemon wedge, or feeling thirsty when absorbed in a story about a hot dry hike with no water show a child how malleable her perceptions and experiences can be.

Stephen Lankton (2006) describes how he targets "chunking logic" as a way to introduce variability with clients. Chunking logic, he wrote, is a term that explains how people take information and use it to make meaning out of their experiences. In the case of depressed or anxious people, the chunking is done in a predictable and not-so-helpful way. Depressed people will "chunk" their experiences through their negative lens. Anxious people might chunk their experiences through their threatening or catastrophic view of their world. Lankton (2006, p. 36) uses "the malleability of perception that is amplified in hypnosis" as a way to reinforce the destabilizing homework assignment: asking clients to select words that will magnify the importance of positive experiences and minimize the importance of negative ones. "Clients learn directly and indirectly that their perceptions are malleable, increasing their sense of ability to choose how they will consider the events that take place in their lives" (p. 36).

How might we teach this to children? The goal is to create an experience that illustrates how perception is variable and how perception can have an impact on how they feel and react, and what they conclude about the events in their lives. With children who are rigidly pessimistic, for example, I ask them to come up with a phrase describing an incident that might happen at school—something annoying or irritating and on the surface undeniably negative: "I slipped on a mustard packet in the cafeteria and dropped my ice cream." We then continue with the tale, making it as positive or silly or preposterous as we can, using those "magnifying" positive words that Lankton described. "Then my ice cream flew through the air and landed in the mushy green beans, and all the kids cheered wildly and called me a hero and we laughed so hard that for the rest of the day my face was stuck in a huge smile. . . ."

How is this hypnotic? Because we are seeding. It is followed by suggestions (either in a formal session or a more casual conversation) that reinforce the shift and can pave the way for future sessions dealing with rigid or negative thinking:

Isn't it interesting, even as we're being silly and playing this game . . . to notice how we can learn something . . . how we turned our words in a different direction . . . how you can start off feeling low . . . and end up laughing. . . . Dropped ice

*cream can be all sorts of things . . . depending on how it lands
. . . and you're learning that sometimes it's okay to step out
of the bad and into the good . . . out of the horrible, terrible,
lousy . . . and toward the hilarious, ridiculous, funny. . . . Not
everything is funny, of course . . . but when you give yourself
a chance to look . . . sometimes you find it . . . the moments
of funny . . . the reasons to smile or giggle . . . and it can help
brighten a difficult day . . . if you give yourself a chance to
look. . . .*

I've given children the assignment of asking several adults or friends their favorite ice cream flavor or favorite color. Predictably they return with many different favorites on the list, prompting me to observe, "Wow, favorite means different things to different people, doesn't it? You have ten different favorite flavors [colors] here! Sometimes we forget what *we* really like is not what someone else likes or enjoys." I've taken out a set of beautiful colored pencils and we have each chosen our five favorites and put them in order of preference. (I make sure my choices are somewhat different than the child's.) Asking a child of any age to tell me about something she used to dislike but now loves, or used to love but now dislikes, is another way of demonstrating variability of experience.

Remember that many children and teens benefit from some guidance or explanation that connects what you are doing together to the broader goals of treatment (Yapko, 2012). For example, in the previous case of demonstrating that experience is variable, a simple statement to a younger child might be, "It's fun to see how you and I and other people have different favorites or ideas about things. Sometimes we get stuck in how we think about things or feel things, but you're learning how you change and grow." More specifically, you might say, "When I first met you, you told me you hated being away from your mom, but I think I see that changing a bit.

. . . You can change, can't you? Just like you changed the color of your bedroom when you grew out of it last year." With older children: "I gave you that assignment to list four things you loved when you were in fourth grade that seem silly to you now. Any idea why? Yes, that's it! I want you to notice *how* much you change your thinking about things. Perhaps when you feel stuck in your anger, that's a helpful memory to have." These statements can be made in or out of trance, but your goal is to deliver them hypnotically. Allow yourself to become absorbed for a moment in the many ways you could do that. . . .

In summary, hypnosis has been shown to be effective with conditions that involve altering one's perceptions, such as traumatic memories and dysfunctional pain (Gfeller & Gorassini, 2010). The list of childhood and adolescent struggles that are helped by such a shift in perception, an alteration in sensation, or a more flexible response is long indeed, and encompasses both physical and emotional symptoms (see e.g., Kuttner, 1988; Anbar, 2001a, 2001b, 2002; Kohen, 2010; Rutten, Reitsma, Vlieger, & Benninga, 2013; Gulewitsch, Müller, Hautzinger, & Schlarb, 2013; Iserson, 2014).

Define the Frame: Questions to Ask Yourself About Variability

Are the child and family flexible or rigid? Do they view and talk about the problem in a rigid or flexible way?

- "She's always been this way, since the day she was born. This type of thing runs in our family. I think she's just wired this way." (rigid)
- "It comes and goes depending on what's happening in her life. Sometimes it's noticeable, but other times she copes very well." "This is new. We haven't seen this before." (flexible)
- "We never do the right thing with him." "He hasn't learned anything from the other therapists we've talked to." "We haven't

found that one answer we're looking for yet." "If he would do what he's told, there wouldn't be a problem." (rigid)

- "We're willing to try anything." "I know there are many opinions about how to handle this issue." "We've done a lot of experimenting over the years, and some things have worked well for a time." (flexible)

The Value of Parts

Please complete these three mental exercises for me:

1. As quickly as you can, list five things that you successfully do (or have done) that require steps to complete (e.g., build a house, cook your award-winning chili).
2. Describe three different roles you have in your life currently, and one former role that for whatever reason you've moved on from.
3. Imagine that you have a difficult ethical question to resolve. Whom do you ask for help? Whose advice do you ignore? What experiences of your own do you draw upon? What unhelpful thoughts do you dismiss?

As you just answered these questions, you took a whole and broke it into parts. The first question required you to think about the sequencing of a larger task, and reminded you of each individual step. To answer the second question, you stepped back and compartmentalized your whole self into different roles, some that you maintain and one that's no longer necessary. The third required you to determine what would be of help, and what to ignore. These skills make up our second important framework of treatment, the importance of parts. All represent a shift away from helplessness, passivity, and global thinking, dangerous patterns that, as discussed earlier, puts kids (and adults) at risk for depression, anxiety, social difficulties, and other problems (Mitchell, Newall, Broeren, & Hudson, 2013; Yapko, 2001, 2009; Seligman, 1995; Nolen-Hoeksema, Wolfson, Mumme, & Guskin, 1995; Kaslow et al., 1992).

Sequencing

Have you ever taught a child to tie his shoes? Dress himself? Socks need to be put on before shoes, underwear before pants. I recently gave my 16-year-old son his first driving lesson. We sat in the driveway, sequentially moving through the steps. First, adjust your seat and mirrors. Then fasten your seat belt. Put the key in the ignition, turn it to start the engine, look behind you, put your foot on the brake, and shift into reverse. And so it went.

Sequencing is familiar to children. They are consistently learning how to move forward, step by step, as they develop new skills. (The goal of this book, as you'll recall, is to provide you a sequence for creating and delivering hypnotic interventions.)

But what happens when the ability to sequence is missing or discarded? The global language of being overwhelmed, not knowing what to do next, or jumping too far ahead into the unknown future shows up. Eighteen-year-old Bethany arrived for her appointment in tears as she talked about going off to college. She worried about picking the wrong classes and the wrong major, making new friends, and even about the job she would get when she graduated. Her mother had the same pattern, calling or e-mailing me frequently about her global concerns for Bethany's far-off future: "I just want her to be able to live comfortably and support herself as an independent adult, whether she gets married or not."

Bethany needed some reminders about the steps involved in the whole process of graduating from high school and moving on to college. I might have told her—as she sat in front of me wiping her tears—that she was capable and smart, had come this far, and could handle not knowing exactly what was next. All helpful things to say, and things that her parents and friends and teachers had likely said to her a lot lately. Knowing she needed more than reassurance, I decided to focus this capable but overwhelmed girl on the framework of sequencing. As you read the following excerpt from the session, notice how being hypnotic adds to the strength of the sequencing message—and sets the stage for the homework to come.

> *I want you to sit back and just exhale a few times, Bethany. Give your-self a moment to settle in internally. . . . Take a few easy breaths. . . . You've been working so hard lately . . . getting so much done . . . big things and small things, inside and out . . . and you can remember telling me about your swim meet last week . . . the exciting story that unfolded . . . race by race and even stroke by stroke . . . second by second. . . . There was an order to things . . . and amidst the excite-ment . . . your friends reminding each other to take it a lap at a time . . . and even now as I'm talking to you . . . noticing another order . . . letting your breath slow down, then your heart rate, then your tears . . . and you know from our experiences together that I'll move from the beginning . . . into the middle . . . maybe with a story about the new recipe I tried last night . . . and then a reminder, directly stated, of how paying attention to the order of things sometimes keeps us moving along . . . and it's the experience of taking steps when we're faced with big projects . . . that helps break it down . . . like a recipe . . . part by part. . . .*

This session, and those that followed, helped Bethany access the past ways in which steps and sequences helped her succeed and allowed her to imagine using those skills again in the future. College, I wanted her to recognize, was not just some big, undefined concept floating in front of her. She would "do college" the way she did swim practices, wrote papers, and cleaned her messy bedroom: a step at a time.

Yapko (1988) described an exercise called the Flow of Steps, in which large, more globally defined goals ("I want to be happy") are broken down into concrete steps. The assignment is to start with a routine event, such as getting a driver's license or swimming at a meet, and identify the many steps involved in accomplishing that goal. I gave Bethany this assignment as a follow-up to our session as a way to help her concretely experience the steps of moving forward. She chose the task of putting a toddler to bed, a familiar babysitting sequence. After doing this successfully, the need for sequencing (and the problems created when she thought about everything at once) became apparent.

Think for a moment about the many global or abstract presenting problems that would benefit from this exercise. For example:

- "I want more friends" or "I don't have any friends."
- "I want to have fun at summer camp" or "I can't handle summer camp."
- "I hate school" or "I wish I did better in school."
- "I'm afraid of dogs" or "I want to get a dog."

The goal is to remind children about the steps they take in everyday life, and activate the use of that template to solve problems and accomplish larger goals.

Compartmentalizing

Compartmentalizing overlaps with sequencing, as it also involves breaking things down into manageable chunks. Compartmentalizing helps children manage their time, their emotions, their relationships, and the demands of the external world. When we teach a child to compartmentalize, we are showing her how to step back, evaluate, and organize herself and her experiences. In more sophisticated language, we are saying to a child: "There are many different aspects and parts of you [or an experience]. You can learn to choose which part of you will work best in this situation or which part of this experience needs your attention."

A child can be taught how to compartmentalize by externalizing, or taking out a part of himself (e.g., worry, anger, impulsivity, stubbornness) and having a look at it. This concept of parts is not new. Virginia Satir used "parts parties" with families; Gestalt therapy has the empty chair; mindfulness practice has the observer. Helping a child name and externalize his "worry part" or obsessive-compulsive part is an effective treatment approach that moves the child out of worried content and into problem-solving mode (Chansky, 2004; March, 2007; Wilson & Lyons, 2013). Rather than a child seeing himself globally as bad, scared, or out of control, he can address the part of him that needs to shift (or get called into action). It's a critical first step when treating anxiety disorders, and I discuss it in much greater detail in Chapter 6.

Compartmentalizing helps to teach boundaries. How we behave or talk in the church compartment, for example, is different than how we behave in the playground compartment. Asking a child to imagine stepping into a different compartment of his life, with different expectations, rules, or roles, allows him to develop the flexibility needed to adapt to change.

Life is full of compartments, so conveying this skill—even to young children—is simple and fun. Examples of compartments abound: in dresser drawers, classes at school, rooms in houses, and pockets in backpacks. Trevor, a 7-year-old boy whose learning challenges often resulted in frustration followed by destructive behavior at school, talked about his compartments in terms of superheroes. When he was just being a regular kid, he was like Clark Kent or Peter Parker. On the monkey bars he was Spiderman. And when he was very angry and out of control, he was the Hulk. Being Hulk during school was not working out well. Peter Parker (who still had the strength and agility of Spiderman) had to learn to think and plan, a much better part of himself to bring to school and activate when he needed to problem solve.

Trevor had a small Spiderman action figure. With permission, he was allowed to keep it handy in his desk or pocket. We rehearsed how to connect to this part of him when he had to read at school, a predictable trigger.

> So let's just imagine, Trevor, that it's time to take out your read-ing book . . . or to go see Mrs. Doyle [the reading specialist].
> . . . Can you imagine that? . . . And maybe some Hulk feelings start to show up. . . . That's okay. . . . We know why. . . . But you have another superhero compartment, don't you? . . . And when you take Spidey out of your desk, or out of your pocket . . . and look at him, you can remember that part of you. . . . Spidey had some struggles, too, didn't he? . . . He had to figure out how to use his powers. . . . You told me it took some time. . . . Can you imagine walking down to Mrs. Doyle's room, you and your Spidey part together? . . . I wonder what you'll think about as you walk . . . walking a step at a time, and reading a step at a time . . . with Spiderman in your pocket.

Using compartments also gives kids a way to talk about aspects of themselves that might feel overwhelming or even shameful. Instead of being told that he was acting inappropriately or needed to calm down, Trevor was able to talk about Spidey and Hulk, which led to conversations about the feelings compartments and how to manage his many emotions.

Connecting and Disconnecting, Signal Versus Noise

The last part of the parts frame focuses on the ability to differentiate between what requires attention and what doesn't. Hypnotically, we may describe it in terms of connection and dissociation. "What shall

I become absorbed in (connected to) and what shall I move away (dissociate) from?" A child can learn to ask herself, "Is this something I need to pay attention to, or can I let it go? Is this a signal or is this noise?" The "something" in question may be external, like the gossip of mean girls at school (noise to ignore), or internal, like a body saying, "Hey, you're tired! Get off your phone and get some sleep" (signal to acknowledge).

This helpful skill enables a child to develop mastery as she learns to sort through the internal and external data of her experiences, and then determine how to respond or react. Children with obsessive-compulsive disorder (OCD) can learn to disconnect from their intrusive OCD thoughts. Depressed children can connect to the positive input they tend to (dis)miss ("Hey, I am good at making people smile"), while distancing themselves from less helpful impulses ("I want to bolt right now, but I can step away from that feeling for a bit"). Children in medical settings can dissociate from discomfort or connect to a pleasant memory. Athletes and performers can shake off a mistake, and focus on what's next and what adjustments to make.

The critical process of connecting to and accessing resources falls into this category, including internal resources ("What do I have inside that can help me here? What will help me handle this?") and social support ("I can ask for help. I know who to talk to about this").

So when should you focus on connection, and when is dissociation or disconnection the right message? Again, knowing the specific message you need to convey within the larger framework is the tailoring that makes for better interventions. Let's look at examples of two similar situations that required very different approaches.

Kendall, age 10, had an emergency appendectomy. A healthy, energetic girl, she had had no significant medical issues and had never been admitted to a hospital before. Everything that led to her surgery happened quickly and with urgency, but happily all went well. She recovered easily and was able to return to her regular activities soon after the surgery. However, Kendall became increasingly focused on her abdomen, worrying about any sounds she heard or sensations she experienced. Even the normal gurgles and growls of hunger and digestion resulted in extreme concern, an unwillingness to go to school, and a demand that she be taken to her pediatrician "just to make sure" she was okay.

Lizi, age 16, was diagnosed with juvenile diabetes when she was 6. Since then, she and her parents had worked diligently and successfully to manage her illness. Each summer since age 10, Lizi attended diabetes camp where she enjoyed a mix of education, camaraderie, and fun. There were few complications and overall she enjoyed good health. Recently, however, Lizi was becoming more lax in her self-care. When her parents expressed their concern, she dismissed them, saying she was on top of things. Knowing she was soon to start driving, her parents were worried that their previously responsible daughter was becoming uncharacteristically careless, a stance that a diabetic teenager couldn't afford to take.

Think about Kendall and Lizi for a moment. In the realm of connection and disconnection, what might you target and introduce?

Kendall, following her surgery, has become too connected to her body, focusing on every sound her tummy makes and treating the smallest of noises as serious alarms. She needs help moving past an experience that was scary but no longer needs to control her. We need to create some distance by helping her put the surgery (and her overreaction to her normal tummy noises) over there so she can focus on what she needs to learn and do as a 10-year-old right here. Part of her session might go something like this:

Kendall, I want to talk to you about something that happened to me, because it reminds me of something that happened to you. . . . A long time ago . . . when I went away to college . . . I moved to the middle of a big city for the first time . . . and at first it was hard to fall asleep. . . . My ears and my brain were listening to everything. . . . My ears and my brain had to learn how to ignore the normal noises of a city night . . . the sirens, the traffic, the beeping of the horns . . . sometimes the construction vehicles that were working below. . . . I had to learn to fall asleep in a different way . . . with different sounds around me . . . and soon I was able to fall asleep. . . . And living in that city . . . I noticed another funny thing, too, when I would walk through the park on my way to school. . . . the French people taking pictures of squirrels . . . normal, regular squirrels. . . . I didn't even notice those squirrels . . . but they don't have squirrels in France. . . . The French visitors had never seen them before . . . and I wondered how long a French girl would have to live in Boston before she started to ignore the squirrels. . . . Just like a country girl had learned to adjust to the noises at night . . . and we all have to make adjustments, don't we? . . . Knowing what's important and what we can ignore . . . what's silly and what's important. . . . We all have different lists . . . depending on how old we are or who we are or where we live . . . and you might be wondering why I'm telling you about alarms and squirrels . . . or maybe you already have an idea. . . . What I want you to hear now is how helpful it is to know what's okay, what's normal . . . and what needs your attention. . . . When your appendix needed to come out, it certainly did a great job of letting you know that, didn't it? . . . and everyone knew that was a signal . . . so you listened loud and clear . . . way back then . . . and it's time now to notice, just for a minute, the quiet noises that are a part of everyday life, like squirrels in Boston . . . or growls in your tummy . . . and even all the other regular things a body does as it grows and eats and digests . . . and if there's another signal . . . you'll know what to do, won't you? . . . Because you can really learn to know the difference. . . .

Lizi, in contrast, has spent 10 years paying close attention to her body, learning how to monitor herself in a very detailed way, something she must do in order to manage her diabetes. Now, though, as she moves toward adulthood and wants her freedom, she is disconnecting from her diabetes and from her body's demands, the opposite of what she needs to do as she seeks her independence. Lizi needs help understanding that a disconnection from her own body can't be included in her quest for independence; in fact, paradoxically, it's quite the opposite: independence through remaining connected to her body. The need to connect to her body as she gets her driver's license and starts planning for a move to college in a few years is even more important as she matures.

For Lizi, the hypnosis session would focus on . . .

all the things that need more attention when you leave the nest. . . . How you have to take care of your car, adding not just gas but oil and windshield wiper fluid . . . and paying attention to the subtle things like alignment and brakes . . . and the details of money and checking accounts and taxes. . . . And if you get your own kitten or puppy . . . the visits to the vet for shots and checkups . . . and how good that can feel . . . to be in charge. . . . But it requires a different level of focus . . . one you've been training for in many ways . . . for many years . . . responsibilities that are added as kids grow and parents can let go . . . and without adults to pick up the slack . . . you get to do your own grocery shopping . . . but also have to make your own meals . . . and the risk of being disconnected . . . might mean an empty gas tank or bank account . . . but you, Lizi, have the advantage of already knowing the risks . . . how to connect to what's important . . . even when it's inconvenient . . . even when you don't feel like it . . . of paying attention to the warning signs . . . the signals . . . and maybe sometimes you'll enjoy ignoring what doesn't matter right now . . . like

the recycling that needs to go out . . . or the alarm clock on a
lazy Sunday . . . or the text from your mom that can wait a bit.
. . . But that's the important part, isn't it? . . . Knowing the dif-
ference . . . and staying connected to you and your body . . .
when it matters. . . . And it matters, doesn't it?

Define the Frame: Questions to Ask Yourself About Parts

Is the problem described as big and overwhelming (global) or more specific (compartmentalized)? Can the child or parents clearly state the issue, the reason for the meeting? Is the problem contained in one aspect of life, or is it more pervasive?

- "We have no idea what's going on. He just seems angry all the time. Nothing we do makes him better." "She's just not herself, and she doesn't know why." "I just feel bad a lot. My life is rotten." "I don't even know where to start!" (global, overwhelming)
- "I am terrified that she'll never learn to relate well to her peers." "This has devastated all of us. How does a family recover from something like this?" "I'm beginning to believe there's something horribly wrong with me." (global)
- "I worry a little during the day, but at night when I try to sleep is when it's a real problem." "She does great when she's performing on stage, but when she has to talk one-to-one, she can't handle it." "She was fine until we separated 3 months ago, and since then she is spending more time in her room alone and her grades are falling." "I can talk to my mom and my friends, but when I talk to my dad we end up yelling." "I have to have surgery on my knee and I want to use hypnosis to handle it better." (specific, compartmentalized)

What does the family focus on, and what do they ignore? What resources already exist in this family? Are they aware and connected to their resources or strengths? What's missing?

- "Our family has been through a lot, so we know how to tackle problems." "She's such a bright kid. She gets great grades in school and has some nice friends." "She has . . . [a sense of humor, imagination, determination, warmth, etc.]" (connected to resources)
- "We don't know what to do. Problems seem to follow us." "She just struggles so." "We've tried so many things, and nothing ever works for long." "Her teachers think she's doing better, but I just don't see it." (focus on weakness, lack of resources)

What value does the child or family put on social connection? Is the child or family engaged socially? Are there friends and activities?

- "He spends a lot of time alone." "He's very shy. He's quiet and keeps to himself." "I wish I had more friends but I'm not good at making them." "All the kids in my class are jerks." (disconnection)
- "I've talked to my girlfriends about this and they have the same issues at home." "He seems happy at school, but miserable when he's home." "She has a boyfriend, but I worry about how she'll handle that." "My best friend is Ben." "I'm having a big birthday party. Lots of my friends can come!" (connection)

Action Counts (Hypnosis Says Do!)

The third and final frame appears at first glance to contradict what most people mistakenly see as the defining feature of hypnosis itself, namely that someone under hypnosis is passive and even willing to be controlled. In truth, action is both a part of the hypnotic experience itself—especially with children—and a critical message we want to convey: Do something! Be a problem solver. Get involved in your own well-being.

Doing hypnosis with children can actually create an active experience where autonomy is heightened—not forfeited. Your suggestions and interactions encourage action, exploration, and engagement out there in the world. Particularly with younger children, these actions and explorations occur right there in the session. This movement (on multiple levels) is exactly what children struggling with depression, anxiety, medical treatment, school, peer relationships, or family issues need. Benjamin, for example, was working on speaking to people outside of his immediate family. His selective mutism made it difficult for him to be independent in virtually all areas of his life, and as a 9-year-old this was annoying him. In our session, he first practiced imagining himself ordering his dinner at a restaurant, and then continued his practice on his own for a few days before going out to eat. After he succeeded he told his mom, "When she asked for my order, I remembered doing what I did in my mind before, and then I did it!"

Depressed children are often stuck in a frame of passivity, frustration, and helplessness. Worried kids lack problem-solving skills and depend on avoidance to keep their anxiety at bay. When we help kids focus upon and engage in the areas of their lives that are changeable and controllable (Hopko, Magidson, & Lejuez, 2011; Wisdom & Barker, 2006), we shift them away from the belief that they have no control and toward a frame that advocates action with positive outcomes. Mood improves, energy increases, and motivation can get a bit of traction. This is the behavioral activation model (Lejuez et al., 2001; Lejuez, Hopko, Acierno, Daughters, & Pagoto, 2011), and although research specifically with children is lacking, it fits rather intuitively with hypnosis. Positive suggestions and experiences in hypnosis combined with positively reinforcing behavioral assignments amplify the message that what you do matters and makes a difference (Yapko, 2010c; Rosen, 1982).

Seligman (1995) describes the importance of contingency or controllability of events beginning in infancy and continuing through a child's development. The awareness of the connection between action and outcome builds a sense of mastery and competence. Babies throw their spoon from their high chair and watch us pick it up so they can throw it again. When my nephew was a toddler, he would repeatedly and dramatically pretend to choke, making his nervous mother come running every time. He was learning cause and effect, and how his actions played out in his world.

Thus, Seligman argued that attempting to build a child's self-esteem by helping her feel special, regardless of what she does, actually makes a child feel worse. Esteem is improved (or worsened) as a measure of one's effectiveness in the world. "Once a child becomes active and hopeful," he wrote, "her feelings of worth always improve" (Seligman, 1995, p. 34).

Baker urged caregivers of children with cancer to "emphasize activity and limit enforced passivity and immobilization," with a "focus on 'turning passive into active'" (1983, p. 79). When this drive for movement and engagement stops or is missing, you must help reactivate it. Problem solving, trial-and-error learning, and the development of autonomy all require some type of action. Focusing on the importance of doing in your hypnotic interventions is essential in many contexts with children.

An active stance involves using a session to rehearse a future event (either imaginatively or actively) and then connecting the rehearsal to a homework assignment or future experience. A child can imagine and practice how she will handle a procedure, sink a foul shot, raise her hand in school, or talk to herself when stressed. Another focus, particularly with anxious children, may be the importance of determining when to stop preparing and start doing. When have you studied enough? Practiced enough? Asked enough questions?

This focus on action is both curative and preventative, and you are sure to discover its value over and over again. As Aristotle said, "For the things we have to learn before we can do them, we learn by doing them."

Define the Frame: Questions to Ask Yourself About Action

Are the problems and the attempts to deal with them described in active or passive language? Do they see the problem as arriving out of nowhere or is there a cause-effect perspective? Do they see it as something they are doing or something being done to them?

- "We don't know what to do. We're hoping you can fix things." "There must be an answer out there somewhere." "Nothing we do seems to make a difference. We give up." "I don't know how this happened." (passive)
- "I am ready to do something about this." "I read about this problem and have some ideas about what to do." "I've been looking forward to this appointment so I can get to work on this." "I can tell you how (when, why) this got worse recently." "I had this problem when I was a kid, but I didn't get help, so we're here to get a head start." (active)

The goal of your intervention may be specific and situational (helping a child manage a medical procedure), or broader (helping develop better emotional regulation). No matter where you start, keep in mind that you have the opportunity to teach children coping strategies both precise enough to address the presenting problem and universal enough to apply to future challenges (Kohen et al., 1984).

If a child is afraid of fire drills, he can learn specifically to tolerate loud noises, but he's even better served by learning to say more broadly, "Unexpected noises (and other unexpected things) will happen. I may not like them, but I can handle them." When a 10-year-old learns to handle the uncertainty of sleepaway camp, she can then generalize this learning to the uncertainty of, for example, her first high school relationship years later. A child that views herself as globally "dumb in school" because of struggles with math may benefit from a new frame that helps her recognize the variety of her strengths and weaknesses, in school and out. A parent that describes her child's anger as the inevitable "family curse" may require interventions that suggest the importance of malleability, learning new skills, and breaking free of not-so-helpful family traditions.

Showing a child how to broaden frames and options in this larger way becomes the gift that keeps on giving, and transcends the particulars of any diagnosis, procedure, or setting. George Eliot, the (female) writer of the late 1800s, said it well: "It is a narrow mind which cannot look at the subject from various points of view."

CHAPTER *5*

Delivering the Session

*H*ow many different recipes exist for chocolate chip cookies? How many varieties and combinations of ingredients? Even if we eliminate the outliers and narrow it down to chocolate chip cookies that actually contain chocolate chips, require some baking, and are in the reasonably accepted size and shape of cookies, there are certainly more variations than a single person could ever bake in a lifetime, and probably many we wouldn't even care to attempt.

What's the point of my cookie analogy? There are as many different possible hypnotic interventions as there are chocolate chip cookie recipes. Because hypnosis with children requires that you tailor the session to fit the needs of the child in front of you, no two sessions could, or should, ever be exactly the same. Similarly, as a baker committed to your craft you should be continually improving your cookie recipes as your skills and knowledge base expand.

Nonetheless, even among the variety, common elements exist

in chocolate chip cookie baking—and in hypnosis. With cookies, a bunch of ingredients are combined, the mix is divided into small portions, and the portions are put into a device that is pretty darn hot for some period of time, and removed to cool when considered done or baked.

Likewise, common elements exist when doing hypnosis with children. In this chapter, I give you a template or recipe for a hypnotic intervention based on the structure given to me by Michael Yapko when I went to my first hypnosis training in 1994 and also described in *Trancework* (Yapko, 2012). As a beginning student of hypnosis, I appreciated (and still do) a step-by-step guide that structured my thinking and gave me a plan. As you will discover, however, children don't care about the structure, the steps, or the elements, and your actual sessions, in real time, will be more like a deliciously baked cookie than an arrangement of carefully measured ingredients.

1. Introduction to Hypnosis
2. Induction
3. Building a Response Set
4. Delivery of the Intervention or Suggestions (Based on Identified Frames)
5. Checking In
6. Posthypnotic Suggestions
7. Closure and Reorientation
8. Seal the Deal: Homework

INTRODUCTION TO HYPNOSIS

Whether or not you discuss the procedure and elements of an upcoming hypnosis session with a child and parents depends on several factors, the most important being the expectations of the child and the parents, your role, and the circumstances of the session. Do you and the families you treat see hypnosis as a separate and distinct part of your practice? Will hypnosis be woven into your treatment of a child's anxiety or behavioral issues, or is there a benefit to defining hypnosis as a distinct skill to be connected to distinct situations, such as during a medical procedure? Will there even be an opportunity for a discussion, or will the hypnosis be spontaneous? This is truly a matter of preference and practice setting.

When I introduce hypnosis, I do a quick and informal talk so a child and parents know generally what to expect. This type of conversation can occur when you meet a child for the first time and the agreed-upon purpose of the meeting is a hypnosis session (for example, a teen calls looking for hypnosis to deal with test anxiety) or when you decide within a session to introduce a hypnotic process as part of the treatment (you're going to incorporate hypnosis to help with an ongoing sleep or anxiety issue). Children and their parents may have questions about how hypnosis works or may wish to share what they have seen or heard about hypnosis.

Kohen and Olness (2011) use the analogy of setting the table to describe this "preinduction." The child is told simply and concretely what will happen in sequence. As you describe the process, use language that orients a child toward positive expectations, introduces a future focus, and includes some posthypnotic suggestions about success. The goal is to make any pretalk a part of the whole treatment experience in a way that builds positive expectancy toward experimentation, change, possibility, and curiosity.

> *I'll ask you to find a comfortable position, whatever works for you. . . . Feel free to try a few out if you'd like. . . . (experimentation, change)*
>
> *So I don't know if you've done this before. . . . So you might be curious. . . . I'll be curious to hear what you think about it. . . . (curiosity, expectancy)*

I love showing kids how to really focus and get absorbed . . . like watching a movie that's so interesting or entertaining that you don't even know time is passing . . . so my words can join your imagination . . . and it's cool to see what can we do to help [name the problem]. (expectancy, possibility)

For an older child or teen who is expecting hypnosis, and even waiting a bit impatiently to begin, your introduction might be like this:

So in a moment, we'll begin. I'll start talking and you'll start listening. You'll probably notice a change in my voice. I might talk a bit slower and even a bit quieter. Your eyes can be open or closed, or both. I'll say something like, "Now go ahead and take a nice breath, and let yourself settle in. . . ." And as I talk and you listen, you might hang on my every word, or you might drift off a bit at times, or you might wonder why I said something . . . or even just ignore me for a bit. At some point, I'm going to check in with you, ask you how you're doing and what you might be thinking about. You can talk to me then, or actually you can talk to me whenever you'd like. After I check in, you'll go back into your focused state for a bit longer. Feel free to adjust your body anytime you need to. . . . If you have an itch, scratch it! You can move around, shift, find what works, get comfortable. When we're done, I'll ask you to open your eyes again and become fully alert and aware, like you are now. If I notice anything interesting along the way, I'll just ask you about it. How does that sound? When we're done we'll talk about what we did and what happens next.

Younger children often have no experience with hypnosis, or don't even know the term. Thus the words you use to describe the experience should maximize what you are hoping to accomplish with the particular child in front of you. In a situation where the hypnosis is more spontaneous or informal, as it often is with younger children and certainly may be with older children as well, you might say:

> *You have such a great imagination. I wonder if we can try something together. Can we use that imagination to help us figure out what to do about [problem]? Let's see. Why don't you settle in right here, and I'm going to tell you about something you might be curious to know. You can close your eyes and listen, or keep your eyes on me and listen, whichever makes it easier for you to use that imagination. It's like listening to a story. Are you ready to listen and see what I have to say?*

If I'm going to invite the child to do something more active, like draw a picture, read a book (or create one), act out a scenario with puppets or stuffed animals, dolls, or action figures, then I simply introduce my props and invite the child to join me.

I make it a practice to record sessions whenever feasible. Therefore, I have my laptop computer with me and often show children how it works. Younger children like to hear their own voices, so to prepare we might practice recording and listening to ourselves in a fun way for a few moments. I generally include this as a part of the pretalk. After the first experience, children know that when I reach for my computer, we're going to have this kind of experience and they will spontaneously start to arrange themselves in preparation. (Adults do the same thing.)

When the hypnotic process is spontaneous—as it often is with younger children—opening a computer to record is not possible and would in fact be intrusive. Do what works best, but I highly recommend that you record sessions as often as possible for a few reasons.

First, it's a record of what you did together, and consequently serves as a protection against any misinterpretations or misconceptions of what occurred. I have never had such a problem in my practice, but I have perhaps preempted the issue a few times by routinely offering a recording to a parent who was not present at the appointment, became concerned when the word *hypnosis* was used, or was looking for a conflict with the other parent or me.

More importantly, though, I record the sessions because I believe it's too hard for almost any child to replicate what we did together later and on his own without concrete repetition and coaching. In fact, I feel the same about my adult clients, too. Listening to a recording of a session that promotes and teaches the skills of pain management, falling asleep, moving out of obsessive thought patterns, or handling anger helps reinforce the work. Children enjoy listening to me (and often to their own voices) as they develop their own mastery. I make the suggestion that they will listen for a time as they learn what they need, and soon won't need my voice on the outside because it will become their own voice on the inside. When I do sessions with adults, I suggest they listen but leave it up to them. Some adults choose not to listen; they want to "maintain the magic" of the session because they are getting the results they want. They want to avoid analyzing or critiquing it. I work with children to come up with a listening plan on a case-by-case basis. As a general rule, I keep the parents out of this. They can assist, but not dictate.

When I started doing hypnosis, I recorded sessions onto tape cassettes and handed them to the client. Then I used a laptop computer and recorded the sessions onto my computer (with an application called Quick Voice) and burned the recording onto CDs for my clients. Now, I often e-mail the recordings to a parent's phone or computer, or the child brings an iPod or phone to the appointment and we transfer it over in my office before they leave.

When Milton Erickson said, "My voice will go with you," I don't think even he could have imagined e-mailing an MP3 recording to a 9-year-old's smartphone.

As with any new skill, children benefit from practicing; your voice and words can be used as an anchor of support. Most children I treat appreciate and use a recording when they begin learning how to self-regulate or change their behavior.

"Do I Call It Hypnosis?"

The question of whether or not to use the term *hypnosis* is a tricky one, at least for me. The simplest answer, though not entirely satisfying, is: If it helps in your work with a child or family to use the term hypnosis then, yes; if it gets it in the way, then no. As a clinician, I want to do what best fits the client. I choose to use hypnotic processes, be they formal or not, because they help children in so many ways.

I don't always see the need to identify hypnosis as separate from what we are doing together. It's why I don't have parents or adult clients sign a separate consent form for hypnosis. Simply saying, "You have such a good imagination, and I'd like to show you how to use your imagination to help with [this problem]" is adequate. The terms *visualization, imagery,* or *pretending* (especially with younger children) work well, too.

On the other hand, sometimes using the term hypnosis is helpful—some would even say essential. Researchers Irving Kirsch and Steven Jay Lynn (1997) investigated how our expectations influence what we do, how we respond to something, and our physiology. Kirsch concluded that the expectations created by the word *hypnosis* are exactly what make hypnotic suggestions powerful: "Rather than controlling expectancy effects, we should want to understand and maximize them" (2000, p. 287). Another study found that labeling an induction procedure "relaxation" resulted in a modest increase in suggestibility, but labeling the process as "hypnosis" resulted in a very significant increase in suggestibility (Gandhi & Oakley, 2005). Therefore it seems wise to use the term *hypnosis* with those who view hypnosis as impactful, even people (particularly teens) who may have impressions based on exposure to hypnosis shows. Their curiosity and expectations about this hypnotic experience can and should be utilized. In fact, I have found that teens with negative connotations about psychotherapy actually welcome the opportunity to do something they see as different and powerful, sometimes even rebellious.

When offered, I hope you take the opportunity to promote the value of hypnosis as a therapeutic tool. If students, teachers, and practitioners of hypnosis don't champion its versatility and range of clinical applications, then who will?

INDUCTION

An induction is quite simply an invitation to participate in the hypnotic experience. The goal is to maximize cooperation and compliance with the suggestions that follow (Zeig, 1988). Yapko described the purpose of the induction as a way to guide the person into hypnosis, and to ultimately narrow the focus of attention on particular experiences and thus disconnect from other "competing awarenesses" (2012, p. 302). You certainly appreciate by now that the "inviting" begins much earlier, with your conscious attention to language, rapport building, creating expectations, and seed planting; but with the induction you are "officially" starting the process, formally or informally, by suggesting a shift of focus, position, sensation.

For people who have exposure to hypnosis through popular media, movies, cartoons, and so on, the induction is often what stands out, what defines the experience as unique. Ask a child (or an adult) to "do hypnosis" and they will likely swing an object in front of your face and give commands to "get sleepy." Would it surprise you to learn that the particulars of the induction may be the least important aspect of your intervention? Current research indicates that the type of induction used doesn't influence responsiveness. Studies by Lynn et al. (2002) indicate no difference between the use of permissive suggestions versus direct commands, brief inductions versus long inductions. It doesn't matter. What does matter is that the induction is used as a ritual to increase positive expectancy, an invitation that says, "Something is about to change!" presented in a hypnotic context.

What does this mean for you and the child in front of you? It means that you have the freedom to invite that child into the experience in whatever way you and the child deem best. It also means that you must be able to flexibly respond to what the child does and make adjustments as needed. The particular induction you use might not matter, but children will still have different developmental needs, interests, spans of attention, and levels of engagement.

Younger children don't usually close their eyes or even sit still. They will be active and conversational. Older children and teens might be more willing to sit quietly with eyes closed and participate in the ritual of hypnosis. The content of your induction should connect to the interests or experiences of the child. You can do this by being specific (a child has a baby sister; therefore you talk about how the baby learns through watching and imitating) or more general (you ask the child to remember the last time when it felt like time flew by, and the last time it felt like time was dragging along).

Research by Lynn et al. (2002) also found that directly emphasizing cooperation—while downplaying the expectation or necessity for an altered or trance state—improves responses to suggestions. For some people, too-high expectations of what they were "supposed" to experience in hypnosis created doubt about the effectiveness of the treatment. "Was I even hypnotized? Did I do it right? I'm not sure I was in a trance. . . . What's a trance, anyway?" This will most likely be a factor when working with teens who are anxious, in a setting where the stakes feel high, like learning pain management or preparing for a big test. In such situations, your goal is to normalize the experience and lessen performance-related thoughts like, "I hope I can do this! What if I don't do it right?" and "Did I do it well enough? Will it work for me?" You accomplish this by engendering a sense of familiarity or recognition with the process. Your objective is to move the child toward your suggestions. Confidence and curiosity increase as she begins to say to herself, "Yes, I know what this person means! I recognize that experience!"

An effective induction becomes the invitation that pulls the child in and focuses her attention. You must seek to join with her, ask for or imply cooperation, and frame the experience as both interesting and connected to her known experience.

Compare these invitations offered to a child scared before a blood draw:

> *I'm going to help you handle this blood draw by showing you how to go into a trance/use hypnosis. . . . I have lots of experience with this . . . and I know how much it can help. . . . It's something that works. . . . I know you've never done it before . . . and I'm here to teach you . . . so let's begin by closing your eyes. . . .*

Or:

> *You've probably had the experience of ignoring one thing because you're so interested in something else, like your mom calling you to dinner . . . and you're deep in the world of that great book or video game . . . or maybe you've had the experience of forgetting to do something, like cleaning your room or finishing your homework . . . because it's boring or unpleasant . . . and you may be wondering . . . because I wonder . . . how we forget to think about something here . . . and then enjoy something over there. . . . Hypnosis is another word for shifting . . . and when your imagination cooperates with my words . . . you can have that experience again right here . . . a shifting . . . and that's a place to start . . . a place you already know from books or videos or games. . . .*

Or with a younger child:

> *I remember you telling me about your favorite book . . . and how*
> *your mom reads to you sitting in that big chair . . . and how you*
> *jump right into the story . . . and you don't even notice what's going*
> *on around you. . . . You even forget to blink your eyes . . . that story*
> *is so interesting. . . . You ignore everything but the fun story. . . .*

In each of the three scenarios the words are supportive and invite the child to learn something new, but the second and third examples connect the child to her known world, suggesting that she already has the tools of disconnection by using common words like *ignoring* and *forgetting*.

Inductions with children can and should be short. In my experience with very young children, a phrase or a few sentences are all that's needed to begin the experience of imagining and focusing and playing. You may choose to use a puppet or stuffed animal to help you deliver the invitation. For example:

> *I wonder if you'd like to use your imagination with me to . . .*

> *Let's do something together, okay? This puppet and I want to*
> *show you a way to . . . [needed skill].*

> *Have you ever gotten an invitation to a party? Has someone ever*
> *invited you to come over to play? I am inviting you to do something*
> *interesting with me . . . something you might already know how to*
> *do [like use your imagination, listen to stories, play pretend, draw*
> *on my whiteboard, etc.]. . . . Let's see what we can do. . . .*

> *I have an experiment . . . and I need your help and cooperation.*
> *. . . You told me about the things you know how to do, like read sto-*
> *ries and draw and come up with great adventures with your buddies*

. . . and we can take those things you already know how to do . . .
and we can use them to show you how to . . . [fall asleep in your
own bed, ride the school bus, go to the dentist, etc.].

The promise of a good story is the simplest of inductions (for children of all ages).

I have a story you might find interesting. . . . It reminds me of
you [or your situation]. . . .

Kuttner's (1988) favorite-story technique was developed for use with children under the age of 6 dealing with acute pain and stress, and was tested on children undergoing treatment for leukemia. Using this approach, the clinician asks the child ahead of time about a favorite story, then uses the story during the medical procedure as a vehicle for creating immediate absorption, familiarity, and reframing. This technique also illustrates the blurred lines between induction, trance, and delivery of the intervention with very young children. The induction becomes simply, "Let me tell you your favorite story, like we talked about. . . ." As Kuttner wrote, "The favorite story became both the hypnotic-induction method as well as the framework for and substance of the trance" (1988, p. 294). Metaphors, language, and specific suggestions regarding the procedure are woven into the story. The focus is on suggestions that amplify competence, courage, and accomplishment.

I talk more specifically about creating and delivering stories and metaphors later in the chapter.

More Extended Induction Ideas

Older children (generally starting at ages 8–10) and teens often expect and tolerate a relatively longer induction that gives them the experience of shifting physical sensations, following a directive, or dissociating from time or place. By longer, I mean a few minutes at the most. Children get bored quickly (adults, too) by a drawn-out countdown or progressive relaxation that plods along. I once experienced an induction where the fellow therapist counted down from 100. By the time he got to 92, I was thinking, "Okay, let's go! I'm ready." By 74, I was no longer interested or absorbed in what he was going to say next.

Below I've listed some additional induction ideas to help spark your own creativity. Most are variations on several well-known and often-used ideas.

Squeezing of Fists

Would you like to try something? It's a game of sorts. . . . Make your hands into soft fists and rest them on your lap. Now together let's squeeze our fists tight. Our faces might join in, too! Now let your fingers release and relax. Can you feel the difference? We might feel some warmth or tingles rush into our fingers. Do you feel that? Now let's see if we can squeeze our fists for a few seconds but keep our faces relaxed. Now let those fingers go. Great! Now this time, let's squeeze our fists for a few seconds while we relax our faces . . . and when we let go of our fists, allow your eyes to close and feel that heaviness in your muscles. Just let those fingers sink into your lap as you sink into the chair. . . .

Palm Squeeze

My son told me about this game that creates a floating sensation:

Put your palms together and put them between your knees. Now try to push your knees apart by pushing your palms away from each other, but squeeze your knees together at the same time. Keep trying. . . . You're doing two things at once. (Con-

*tinue for several seconds.) . . . Keep pushing and pulling . . .
and when you stop, you can close your eyes and allow yourself
to float. . . . Go ahead and stop . . . and notice that shift . . .
the tension that floats away. . . .*

Fingernail Face

Draw a little face on the thumbnail of the child (Morgan & Hilgard, 1978).

*Now I want you to hold your arm out in front of your face . . .
and put your thumb up. . . . Give yourself the thumbs up
. . . and see that silly face we drew, looking back at you. . . .
Focus on that face . . . and then let that arm start to move,
as if it's heavy . . . and follow the face as it moves downward
toward your lap . . . just like that . . . and when it gets there,
wherever that may be . . . you can watch that face . . . and
listen to my words at the same time . . . or close your eyes
when you like. . . .*

This can lead to some fun word play with the word *face*, as you talk about what she's learning to face, facing challenges, being face-to-face with what you're learning to face, and so on.

Eye Fixation

*Can you find something to look at, anywhere in this room . . .
a design on my carpet or a word on the bookshelf or spot on
the wall? . . . And you can stare easily, noticing the details . . .
and gaze as perhaps your breathing slows a bit . . . and your
blinking slows a bit. And if you feel your eyelids wanting to
rest, if your eyes need a break from all that looking, you can
allow them to close. . . . It's up to you . . . and as you look with
your eyes . . . open or closed . . . you can see what there is to*

see on the inside, too, what you can look at . . . what you can
examine . . . what you might notice. . . .

Imagining Gravity

You know what gravity is, don't you? As you sit here, maybe
you can imagine that I have a special power, and you do, too.
We can turn up gravity ever so slightly . . . and as we do, you
can feel yourself sinking down a bit into the couch . . . ever
so slightly . . . in such an interesting way. . . . Turn gravity up,
muscles sink down. . . . I wonder who first noticed gravity. . . .
What a discovery that must have been. . . .

Television or Movie Screen

Together we're going to look for ways to manage [the problem].
Maybe we can begin to see some solutions, and see what your
creative brain can come up with, too . . . and you know how
absorbed you can get in a favorite show or movie or video. . . .
So can we imagine you're watching a show? . . . And you're so
absorbed. . . .

From here, the options to tailor the upcoming intervention are
boundless. Does the child enter his favorite show and get help from
the characters? Does he change the channel and create his own show,
starring as the competent problem solver? Does he watch the problem
arise, then hit stop on the remote, discuss a different way of handling
it with you, then hit play and watch the new, reframed outcome?

Early Learning Set

This well-known induction (Erickson, Rossi, & Rossi, 1976, pp.
6–7) recalls for the listener the universal and seemingly "big insur-
mountable task" of learning letters and numbers as a kindergar-

tener, and how the process of learning creates mental images that are now permanent. Rosen (1982) also shared Erickson's story of learning to walk again after his polio by observing his baby sister, explaining the general and positive process of how people learn something new and eventually adopt a skill without needing to think about it consciously.

I adapt this with children as I discuss how

there are so many things you know how to do today that you couldn't do even a year ago, a few months ago, and what if you think about what you learned this year in school, or how you learned to ride a bike, or multiply fractions, or take the bus on your own? . . . And now you do these things, without really thinking much about them, don't you? This is how you learn new things, by watching and doing and practicing . . . until they become automatic. . . . This is how you figure things out. . . .

Confusion

Confusion techniques (Erickson, 1964) involve doing or saying something in an illogical or unexpected way, which results in momentary confusion and a search for meaning. The goal is to interrupt a pattern with words, actions, or suggestions that create an opening for a new perspective (Yapko, 2012; Kohen & Olness, 2011). We might describe such strategies as experiential curveballs: the child expects a more straightforward delivery, but the delivery changes in a way that throws him a bit off balance. Kohen and Olness (2011) noted that these Ericksonian-based techniques are effective with children who are frightened or in great pain, and thus already in a heightened state of focus. For example: "When you scream that loud, I listen carefully. . . . The loud might scare away a bird or a butterfly, but it asks me to get close to where the quiet is . . . where we can start to breathe together like this. . . ."

Wordplay can be used with older children to create memorable interactions. For example, I introduced the use of trance to an anxious teen by saying, "Go inside and focus on your worry . . . your boring, boring worry . . . your worry that likes to say the same thing and do the same thing . . . as predictable as the tide. . . . It comes in waves like sea swells, and when you see sea swells, you can dip under the waves. . . . You don't have to be as predictable as the same old waves of worry. . . . Ain't that swell? . . ." He came into the appointment convinced that his anxiety "showed up out of nowhere" with a goal to "stop it from happening." My words hit him between the eyes with a completely different concept: his worry was boring and predictable (rather than surprising) and there was no need (no way) to stop this natural response (like the waves and the tides), so we needed a new frame.

Previous Experience

If a child has had previous (and positive) experience with hypnosis or any kind of relaxation, meditation, or imagery, simply ask her to "remember that experience, how your body felt, and just allow yourself to take the memories from then, and use them now. . . . Even if you can't remember the details . . . it can be a starting place for us both. . . ." You can also reference any common experience that involves absorption, like becoming absorbed in a good book, or "playing a game with friends that was such fun it made the day fly by. . . ."

The Convincer

There are times when an induction can be presented as a preview of what happens in hypnosis—what I sometimes call a convincer. Earlier I discussed how high expectations of being in a trance state can create performance anxiety in children and parents when the stakes are high and the pressure to "do it right" is heightened. A short process billed as a practice session can help decrease some of this anxiety while building rapport, trust, and confidence. Below is an example of a practice induction that—in a very short amount of time—introduces the child (and parents) to the hypnotic experience, increases a sense of mastery, and paves the way for future sessions. Taking the pressure off with some practice normalizes the process and answers questions experientially. Whatever you call it, remember that this experience is part of the therapy; therefore, don't let it go to waste. The script below is an example of a simple convincer I call Heavy Hands, and it is full of suggestions that seed the work to come.

> *How about sitting right here, with your hands resting gently in your lap or by your side. . . . Let's start by taking a few deep, full breaths. Fill up your lungs like two balloons, and then let the air out easily, in and out of your nose or your mouth. [Do this together for two or three breaths.] You can go ahead and close your eyes if you want to, just to help you relax and focus a bit more, or you can leave them open, too. And let your breathing become smooth and natural, like when you're asleep or just watching TV or a movie. You don't have to think about it. Just let your body do what it knows how to do. In and out, in and out, easy and through your nose.*
>
> *Now I want you to make your face soggy. Have you ever used that word to describe your face? Make all the muscles in your face loose. Just let them hang there. And smiling is okay, too, of course. [Kids often smile here. . . Make it okay for them to do so.] Soggy or smiling, smiling and soggy. . . .*
>
> *Go ahead and put all of your attention onto one of your hands. It doesn't matter which one. You can even choose both if you like. You can pay attention to your hand, even if your eyes are closed. You can be aware of every knuckle and every fingernail. You can feel the temperature of your hand. . . . Maybe the top feels different than the palm. You can notice the texture of the material that your hand is touching. You can notice your thumb and your pinkie, and the fingers in between.*

Now let those fingers begin to feel heavy, bit by bit, heavier and heavier. You can imagine that there is something tied to those fingers, like bricks or pianos or tree trunks, and each of those fingers is sinking down, getting heavier and comfortable. Maybe your fingers will start to feel warm, or a little tingly. You could lift your fingers if you wanted to, because you are in control of your body, but maybe it would be too . . . much . . . work. So you can let them just stay where they are, getting heavier and more relaxed. It's an interesting feeling to create.

And you might notice the heavy, relaxed feeling moving into other parts, too. Maybe your hands, and your wrists, and your arms and shoulders are feeling heavy. And maybe your eyelids feel a bit heavier, too. I wonder what other parts feel comfortable. Your feet? Your toes? Your forehead? Your ears? Only you can know.

Stay here for a bit longer. Let that heavy comfort hang around. And as you notice that heaviness, listen to this: Wherever you are . . . school . . . home . . . falling asleep in bed . . . riding along in the car [fill in other situations here] . . . you can create this feeling of heaviness in your hand, just by taking a few deep breaths and imagining that hand getting heavy. Just by imagining those bricks or those pianos, or whatever you come up with. . . . And when that hand starts to feel heavy, the rest of you, even your brain, can slow down, too. It's as if your hand is the reminder to the rest of your body and your mind. And what can your hand remind you of? What feels good to remember? To create?

The more you practice, the better you'll become at asking that hand to get heavy. You can even do it with your eyes open. You can do it while you're talking to someone. With that one heavy hand, the rest of you remembers how you can create helpful sensations in parts of you, wherever you want to, whenever you want to.

In a few moments, when you're ready, you can start to wiggle those fingers a little, and even wiggle your toes if you like. Your hand and the rest of you can begin to move around a bit, and you can open your eyes [if they're closed]. Take a few more deep breaths, as you feel alert, eyes open . . . and how cool that you just learned to create something in your own body, something that can help in all sorts of different ways. I wonder how you'll use this new power, this new discovery. You might already have some ideas, or maybe it's time to start looking. . . .

BUILDING A RESPONSE SET

You've established rapport, identified a target, and invited the child in front of you on an interesting journey to change the way he thinks or responds. You're ready to head out (or in) together—to have an experience that will create, develop, or strengthen this child's resources.

But wait! There's one more useful step, and it's called building a response set.

The goal of a response set is to increase the likelihood that the child (or any client) will accept the suggestions to come. This is done by building momentum in a responsive direction. By offering general truisms that suggest a new frame—statements that suggest where you're headed and are easily accepted—you gently open the door to the more specific suggestions to come (Yapko, 2012; Lynn, Surya Das, Hallquist, & Williams, 2006; Erickson et al., 1976).

The implicit message conveyed is simply this: "We're going to work on XXX. Therefore I'm going to plant the seeds of possibility by talking about XXX now in a general, unchallenging way."

Milton Erickson frequently described his use of a "yes set" (Erickson et al., 1976; Erickson & Rossi, 1979), a series of statements (truisms) or questions that easily engender a "yes" response. A popular Erickson story (Erickson et al., 1976) describes a student's experience with a resistant client who refused to accept an invitation to go into trance. The student asked the subject 20 to 30 routine questions, all of which required an obvious "yes" response. When the client was finally asked again if he would like to go into trance, he agreed, perhaps to end the boring litany of questions and because "yes" seemed the reasonable next response. (I have come across an article about an attorney who teaches such a "yes set" cross-examination technique. By asking a litany of factual questions that have easy "yes" responses, he believes it makes a witness on the stand less likely to then lie when asked a more pivotal question. He denied having any knowledge of Erickson.)

The yes set is perhaps the most well known, but I encourage you to think about developing responsiveness in versatile ways. Yapko (2012) describes the use of the "I don't know" set, a great way to prime for flexible coping and the tolerance of uncertainty (both critical in the treatment of anxious children). Or how about a response set that talks about discovering old treasures, a helpful idea as you prepare a child to elicit past successes in order to cope with present challenges?

Remember the broad therapeutic frames discussed in Chapter 4? How might you develop a response set for each of these? What truisms would suggest movement toward the activation or development of these perspectives?

The Three Frames

- Experience is variable (vs. rigid and permanent)
- The value of parts (vs. global and overwhelming)
  - Sequencing
  - Compartmentalizing
  - Connection and disconnection, or signals and noise
- Action counts (vs. passive and avoidant)

For example, if I'm working with a child whose rigid framework impedes her ability to handle new or unfamiliar experiences, I want to ultimately convey that change is an inevitable part of growing and learning. I want to suggest in a general way that experience is variable, that increased flexibility is the goal. Statements that normalize change and gently remind her of the many changes she (and most other children) have already handled might sound like this:

- You've certainly learned a lot since you were born (and you can be open to learning more).
- Most kids your age know the moon isn't made of cheese. (You've figured things out as you've matured; your beliefs have changed.)
- I wonder, when I talk to you about things that change . . . I wonder what comes to your mind? . . . The months, the weather, your bedtime, the size of your feet?

With young children, as I've mentioned, you must often be quick and concise. Thus the induction and the response set may overlap. Let's revisit the induction of the young child in need of a blood draw:

> *I remember you telling me about your favorite book . . . and how your mom reads to you sitting in that big chair . . . and how you jump right into the story . . . and you don't even notice what's going on around you. . . . You even forget to blink your eyes . . . that story is so interesting. . . . You ignore everything but the fun story. . . .*

Now add some truisms to build the response set of disconnecting further and then move right into the suggestions:

> *Sometimes we listen, and sometimes we ignore.*

> *You told me you have a dog, didn't you? . . . And I know dogs that come when they're called, but sometimes they ignore their owners when they're chewing a stick or chasing a squirrel. And I know some kids who are good at ignoring, too! Have you ever*

heard of good ignoring? Sometimes one hand ignores the other hand. . . . It's true! You might do it.

You're learning to write your letters and numbers with this hand, right? Sometimes when kids are learning to write with their right hand, or learning to draw shapes or funny faces, they leave the left hand alone . . . just forget about it for a time.

Next, I might offer more direct suggestions about choosing to ignore what's happening on the left, while enjoying what she can write on the right; letting the nurse pay attention to her job, while she gets to pay attention to what she's learning as a child . . . some fun learning and good ignoring.

Later, when she gets her blood drawn, we'll alert the nurse to use the left arm, then give her right hand some paper and colored pencils to draw with, and further engage her by drawing funny faces or practicing her letters together, or having her point out pictures in her favorite book. (But I'm getting ahead of myself here.)

In summary, making the effort to build responsiveness (even when done in a few short minutes or sentences) is a strategic move that increases the success of your interventions (Erickson & Rossi, 1979; Zeig, 2001; Yapko, 2012). Zeig (2001) uses the phrase "doubling up," which reminds us to use every opportunity—from the start—to move toward the therapeutic goal. Challenge yourself to choose words that are connected to the therapeutic goal, and play with building response sets to further enhance your effectiveness.

DELIVERY OF THE INTERVENTION OR SUGGESTIONS (BASED ON IDENTIFIED FRAMES)

You recognize by now, of course, that as you move layer by layer through the process of creating hypnotic interventions, suggestions start immediately, particularly with younger children and in acute

118

settings. As Kohen and Murray (2006) observed, suggestion is an inevitable part of clinical interactions—and of most interactions, actually. With practice and awareness you can use suggestive language fluidly in order to elicit or develop the resources a child needs. Upcoming chapters offer plenty of content examples; here I discuss some broader process considerations including direct versus indirect suggestions, the use of metaphor and storytelling, and the importance of collaboration.

Direct or Indirect?

Suggestions, like inductions, should incorporate the child's language, match the level of development, and have a tone of curiosity and experimentation. The general consensus among practitioners of pediatric hypnosis is that a permissive approach that supports an internal locus of control and amplifies resources is preferable to an authoritative stance, or one that provides scripted content (Kohen & Olness, 2011; Sugarman & Wester, 2013). Better to suggest that a child "explore a safe/fun/interesting/relaxing place" versus the specific instruction to imagine "taking a walk in the woods" or suggesting a child imagine "floating on a cloud." You should aim to incorporate information about the child's interests, but in developing a child's sense of mastery and self-efficacy, we do not want to limit a child's ability "to discover his or her own stories, metaphors, and attributions of meaning" (Sugarman & Wester, 2013, p. 13).

Be careful not to confuse an authoritarian approach with a direct (concrete) approach. It is possible and often necessary to be direct with a child based on a variety of factors, including age and language development, but you can be direct while also being permissive and inviting. For example, if the goal for a child is to acclimate to the fire drills at school and the inevitable startle response that happens (by design), I might suggest directly, "Now we can imagine [or experience] the moment when the alarm rings and what that startled feeling does in your body . . . and then how it fades away. Your body moves from startled back to okay, and that can happen at school, just like we've practiced it here." If I were being authoritarian about it, I'd say, "You will feel startled by the alarm but that feeling will go away quickly."

Using direct language or indirect language is a matter of clinical judgment. The goal is to determine what will work best for the child at any given moment, and this may take some trial and error. Children with Asperger's syndrome, for example, have difficulty with figurative language, metaphors, sarcasm, humor, and implication, and therefore they require a direct, concrete use of language. Many children, including those on the autism spectrum, will benefit from direct suggestions that clearly connect what you discuss in a session with other situations they will encounter in the outside world (D. Yapko, 2006).

Most often, movement between direct and indirect suggestions is the norm, not the exception. I remember directly asking a worried 6-year-old, "Draw a picture of what it looks like in your tummy." She politely said, "No, thank you." Consequently, I shifted my approach: "Sometimes tummies feel strange or nervous, and kids like to imagine what might be going on in there. They use pictures or words, and one girl I know did a dance about her tummy! Some kids draw butterflies in their tummies, and some kids draw faces, and some kids just scribble. I wonder what you might do. . . ." I started to draw a picture of a girl who looked like her. She watched me for a minute and then picked up her own red marker and began to color in the stomach area. The next time she saw me, she walked in and announced, "I am going to draw something for you." A direct communication, indeed.

Here's another example: If I wanted to help a child develop the ability to pause before blurting something out in school, I might start by saying directly but permissively, "Let's practice an easy inhale and exhale, and let's use those few seconds to pause."

After practicing this a few times, commenting on how we are paying attention to this natural thing called breathing, I introduce the idea of connecting this known skill to a new skill:

Breathing in and out is something you already know how to do. . . . You've been doing it since the moment you were born! So we can take this expert skill and connect it to another new skill that needs a bit more practice . . . the skill of pausing. . . . Let's take something you're really good at . . . and use it to practice getting really good at something else. . . . How many seconds can a breath in and out give you? Thank you, breath, for being such an easy pause. . . . How many seconds? Let's count together. . . .

I follow this with an invitation to "come up with your own simple phrase that reminds you how helpful those few extra seconds can be." We practice together, and record our practice, and I then give a concrete instruction to practice at home and in school, getting better and better every time, "because that's how practice works." My instructions are direct, but permissive.

If I wanted to be more indirect, I might say:

I wonder how many seconds it takes to breathe in and breathe out? [Model a slow inhale and exhale.] We talk about holding our breath. When you go under water, you hold your breath, don't you? But I wonder if you could take a breath while you hold something else . . . taking and holding. . . . When we want people to wait, we say, "Hold your horses!" or "Hold your water!" or "Hold that thought!" or even "Hold your tongue!" What expression do you like best? What words could you say to yourself . . . so you could take a breath . . . nice and easy . . .

in and out . . . just like that! . . . But remind yourself to hold on
for a few seconds. . . . What could help you remember? Take a
breath . . . take a moment . . . a moment for you . . . and hold
. . . what? You choose. . . .

Together we want to create a different experience that connects an automatic skill ("take a breath") with some new learning ("hold on . . .") in a bit of a surprising way.

Indirect suggestions come in many different forms, from stories to jokes to puns to questions. Most often, indirection is tied to permissiveness, giving the child options and autonomy, making her the captain of her ship. The goal, as with any suggestion, is to elicit or activate a response, but you are making the request in a less confrontational way, more like sidling up to the situation. The suggestion might be hidden or embedded in a story or a joke, or the language used may "allow" the child to follow your directions without having to consciously "feel" like she is obeying.

Using Stories and Metaphor

Being indirect by using stories and metaphors is often both effective and enjoyable. The children I work with love to hear about the other children I've seen over the years who conveniently had problems similar to their own. Children of all ages engage when a good story is told well. George Burns wrote that the words *once upon a time* "are an invitation into the phenomenon of hypnosis where listeners are entranced, attention is focused, time is distorted, and the client can share the challenges, problem-solving strategies, and goal attainment of the fictional hero" (2006, p. 59).

Stories allow for the creation of flexible solutions and allow for the child to contribute to its ending, thereby personalizing it to make it her own. Anecdotes are memorable, engaging, and surprising, and send a person on a search for meaning and personal applicability (Zeig, 1980; Erickson & Rossi, 1979). Linden described the importance of magic in stories and play "as a way to make things happen that ordinarily cannot happen. It can give children a sense of control and mastery in situations which seem hopeless, and does so with delight and joy. . . . The possibility of magic restores hope" (2003, p. 247). Some evidence suggests children prefer metaphorical language to direct suggestions (Heffner, Greco, & Eifert, 2003). Most important is creating stories and metaphors that are meaningful and attractive to the child (or adult) in front of you (Lankton & Matthews, 2010).

Here are some general guidelines to help you find, create, and deliver effective stories and metaphors to children.

- First and foremost, know your therapeutic target. George Burns (2006) emphasized the importance of knowing from the start the desired outcome of your intervention, and how your story will then illustrate the resources needed to get there, just as I described in detail in Chapter 4. Burns (2001, 2005, 2006) described a PRO (problem, resources, outcome) model for creating therapeutic stories that I find helpful. The story starts by first introducing the Problem (similar to the child's), then describes the skills and Resources needed to address the problem, and ends by describing the Outcome of the story, which mirrors the child's therapeutic goal. I recommend going after a single issue per session or story.
- Begin to collect stories and tales to share with children, focusing on the common skills and resources children and teens need in general, and more specifically with the population you serve. Many resources specific to hypnosis are available (for example, Burns, 2001, 2005; Thomson, 2005) as well as books of fables, teaching stories, and children's literature. I have included an annotated bibliography of children's books that promote flexibil-

ity, resilience, learning, and so on, in Appendix B. I suggest you start your own list as well. Older children relate to current events, historical metaphors, movies, novels, and stories about peers.

- Stories and metaphors can be short and direct. Don't feel intimidated by the need to create tales with hidden meanings or clever messages. With practice and attentiveness, we all can makes significant strides forward. With younger children, in fact, I often simply say, "I have a story about a girl like you who had a problem that reminds me of you." I often change the content a bit, but focus on the process needed to solve the problem at hand.

- Help the child, when indicated, to understand the story and how it connects to her situation. Not all people in the field agree. Kay Thompson wrote, "Don't waste your time telling a metaphor if you are then going to turn around and explain why you told it, because that doesn't really help" (Kane & Olness, 2004, p. 96). I don't have a problem explaining a story, particularly with children. We can hope that our subjects glean the meaning of our stories and metaphors, but if a child misses the meaning of what we're hoping to teach and we aren't there to help him get the meaning, that doesn't help either, does it? I just ask, "What do you think of that story?" or "Do you know why I told you that story?" If the child's interpretation is different than what you intended (but still helpful), then use it. Does the child recognize a different resource? Then amplify it. Conversely, pay attention to what the child doesn't recognize in the story or metaphor. Was the child unable to see the hope in what you intended to be an optimistic story (a likely cognitive pattern in a depressed or catastrophic child)? Did she miss the message that mistakes are a necessary part of learning? That's important therapeutic information you must recognize and then address (Matthews & Langdell, 1989).

- Be collaborative with children. Ask them what they think might solve the problem, or have them predict what the main character will do to get out of the situation. I often present a problem to a child and then ask for help because I have some ideas but I'm a bit stuck. Or, in order to cement the learning and success the child has already demonstrated, I'll ask the child to help me with another (invented) case "because I know you've already handled something like this." I might say, "Tomorrow a girl is coming to see me for the first time, and she is having a terrible time going to school. You have been handling your mornings so well! Can you give me some advice? Is there a story I can tell her that might help?" I find this particularly helpful when kids aren't in the mood to talk about themselves or their issues. As they tell me the story, I model focused attention and absorption in the story. We both go into trance.

CHECKING IN

When I was first learning to do hypnosis with adults, I felt strange checking in with them during the session. What if I "ruined" their experience by interrupting their focus or rudely disturbing them? Adult and teen clients generally sit cooperatively and quietly; consequently, interacting with them seemed intrusive. Many years of experience have taught me three things: first, checking in with clients is helpful, not intrusive; second, a formal check-in with children is rarely necessary because the entire experience is usually more interactive to begin with; and finally, during your quick introduction to hypnosis, you describe this aspect of the experience, and therefore the child (and adult) expect it.

Asking a few simple questions after you have delivered your message confirms that the child understands or allows you to offer more clarification as needed. We want the child to go inside and find the resources needed, but we need to know we've offered enough assistance to hit the mark. There's no benefit to leaving a child confused or disconnected from the therapeutic goal.

I say to a child, "I'm going to check in with you now, just as I told you I would. You can tell me what you've been thinking about . . . or experiencing . . . or you can tell me anything at all. Anything you'd like to share?" Generally children willingly talk, although you may need to wait a moment or two if the child has been sitting still with eyes closed, deeply relaxed or cataleptic. This is your opportunity to ratify new learning or understanding, or to clarify if needed.

If I child doesn't respond to my first request, I check in more directly and ask yes or no questions. "Can you hear the sound of my voice? You can nod yes. Good. If you'd like to talk now, just nod and let me know, and take your time. You might feel very relaxed and comfortable. If you don't want to talk right now, just shake your head no. That's fine too." You may then choose to continue communicating with yes and no questions that can be answered nonverbally with nods, headshakes, or finger raises. "I've been talking to you about [brief summary of suggestions]. I can see you're very focused right now, aren't you? Let me know that you're doing okay with these [ideas, thoughts, stories] by just [giving me a thumbs up, raising your finger, nodding your head a bit]." If the child does not want to communicate much, then acknowledge that and move forward, making the suggestion that the two of you can talk more together when you have brought this experience to a close.

POSTHYPNOTIC SUGGESTIONS

After confirming the message has been adequately conveyed, it's time to solidify the learning. We want to concretely help the child take what she has learned and experienced in the session and apply it to her life outside this experience, a process referred to as contextualization. Posthypnotic suggestions follow a simple format: "When you are in situation XX, you will be able to YY."

Let's return to the example above of a young boy learning to take a pause before blurting out answers in class. The message is one of increased self-control, self-awareness, and better boundaries. The posthypnotic suggestion may begin very specifically:

When you are sitting in class, tomorrow or the next day or any day after that, you can remember what we practiced here and what you've been practicing at home . . . noticing the inhale and the exhale, and how this can remind you to "hold your horses" for a few seconds, wait for the teacher to call on you, or wait for others to finish speaking . . . and that little pause that you know how to do . . . taking a breath while you hold yourself still . . . can allow you to answer . . . to share what you know . . . which feels great inside and out.

The posthypnotic suggestion can then become more generalized, depending on age and developing skill level:

And then in other places, like playing with friends or at soccer practice or even at the dinner table with Mom and Dad . . . you can keep practicing how to take a breath in and out, hold on for a moment when you need to . . . and practice sharing your words and your experiences when the time is right . . . and I wonder how others will notice what you're learning . . . how you will notice you saying to yourself . . . "Take a breath and hold your horses." . . . You might even smile to yourself like you're smiling right now. . . .

It's also smart to make a suggestion for increased success during future hypnosis sessions with you (or in any clinical setting) and success when practicing at home:

And the next time we're together or when you're practicing [your hypnosis skills] at home, you might even discover some- thing very cool . . . that practicing, even for a minute here or

a minute there, can make it easier for you to get focused . . .
to talk to yourself in this different way . . . and handle [specific
situation] in a way that works great for you. . . .

I particularly like making general suggestions to a child for
"future discovery," an age progression strategy that allows for later
connection to the resources created or amplified during a session: "I
don't know and you don't know all the ways you'll use these skills
. . . where or when. . . . It can be fun not to know exactly how you'll
make it happen!" (Yapko, 2012). This can be helpful when dealing
with generalized anxiety, depression, OCD, chronic health issues, or
any other issue that occurs in many different contexts. If the context
of the problem is predictable and specific, then certainly be specific;
but why not also generalize skills whenever possible?

Additionally, I prefer posthypnotic suggestions that are permissive, allow for trial-and-error learning, and promote coping, managing, or reframing of sensations or experiences rather than a promise
of elimination. For example, I prefer the suggestion, "When you walk
into the classroom to take the test, you may notice your body reacting in that familiar way, but you can respond to these sensations differently, because you know so much more about yourself and your
body's reactions." I would avoid a suggestion like, "When you enter
the room for the test, you will feel a sense of calm and relaxation
come over you. No worries, no stress, and you'll be able to think
clearly while you take the test." The upcoming chapters illustrate
how I combine cognitive strategies with hypnosis when dealing with
specific clinical situations.

CLOSURE AND REORIENTATION

Once done with the posthypnotic suggestions, simply bring the
experience to a close by realerting and reorienting as needed. For
older children:

We've talked about many things like [give examples] . . . and so
you can take a moment or two to sort through some new ideas or
interesting words . . . and continue to discover what will be most
helpful or interesting to you . . . and when you're ready you can
open your eyes, feeling refreshed and ready for what's next. . . .

Children who have been sitting with eyes closed or with little
movement (catalepsy) may need a few moments to open their eyes,
stretch their limbs, and reconnect with their surroundings and with
you. As they open their eyes and reengage with me, I usually say
something profound like, "Hi, how're you doing?" They usually say
something like, "Good!" I then process the session briefly, asking a
few general questions. "Is there anything you'd like to share? What
was that like for you? Do you have any questions? What stands out
for you about the experience?"

Younger children who have been active throughout the experience don't need much in the way of realerting, but it's important and
helpful to debrief with them about what they learned, and hear about
any other ideas they may wish to share: "So now you have some ways
to handle XX. Do you have any questions for me? Do you have any
other ideas for me? Is there anything you'd like to share?"

SEAL THE DEAL: HOMEWORK

For most children, practicing and independently using the hypnotic
techniques they've learned is an important next step in the process,
and is typically referred to as self-hypnosis. Gail Gardner, in her 1981
article on the teaching of self-hypnosis to children, defined it this
way:

Children's use of self-hypnosis refers to their ability to experi-
ence hypnosis for explicit therapeutic purposes without the physical

129

presence and direct guidance of another person. . . . The child has had previous heterohypnotic experience, (meaning with another person guiding the child) and a therapist has provided guidance in the use of self-hypnosis. . . . The child's goal is to be able to utilize hypnotherapeutic techniques in his own behalf at any time or place where it would be good to do so, without having to rely on the presence of the therapist. In short, the child masters the skills of hypnosis and enjoys full ownership. (p. 302)

I fully agree with this definition and with the goal. Autonomy and mastery are the linchpins of children feeling capable of changing their own experiences for the better. Teaching a child the skill of shifting her focus, changing the way the body feels, or reacting differently to a thought or situation is what this is all about. But I am also aware of the frequent use of the term *self-hypnosis*, and the routine use of the phrase "all hypnosis is self-hypnosis." Does the routine use of these words diminish the importance of rapport, connection, and support? I'm afraid it might. Although your ultimate goal may be for a child to manage his own asthma, headache, or anxiety, your therapeutic presence and connection—in the office and out—hugely impacts the outcome.

Perhaps it is a matter of semantics, but not all hypnosis is self-hypnosis, for much of the benefit comes from the connection that a child has with you and your voice. You would be wise to acknowledge your impact (Yapko, 2014). Your expectancy, your hope, your attention are powerful placebos in this interactive relationship. You are seeding, modeling, and mirroring. You are checking in and then adapting, thereby giving the message that you and the child are in this together. Even when a child is independently using his self-hypnosis skills—heading onto the school bus or into the lab for a blood draw—your relationship, your voice, is there. And I see that as a good thing.

As I said earlier, I almost always record hypnosis sessions, easier now than when Gardner was writing in 1981. Logistically, recording the full session is easier with older children as the session has a more distinct start and finish; the spontaneous hypnotic interactions with younger children can sometimes make it tricky. Nonetheless, I find it so helpful for a younger child to have a recording for later practice that I often just do a brief 3–5-minute reminder that focuses on the primary target, and refers to the longer talk we had in the office as a way to connect our session with the practice at home.

Before children leave the office, we record something like this together:

> *Do you remember how we talked today about the cool way you imagined leaving your arm with the nurse while you travel off to that funny froggy parade we laughed about? Let's practice that together right now for a minute. . . . Can you remember what we said and what you imagined? [I share a few reminders as needed, but allow the child to describe the process as desired.]*
>
> *That's great . . . and when you are listening to this at home or in the car, you can take that nice breath . . . and close your eyes or leave them open . . . and imagine that fun froggy parade . . . and how you saw the hop hop hopping . . . and how you joined right in . . . and your smile gets bigger while your arm gets looser . . . and you move right along with this silly parade . . . from lily pad to lily pad. . . . Leave your arm over here for a bit so you can hop over there . . . and for five hops you forget your loosey-goosey arm . . . so count the hops inside your imagination . . . or count out loud if you like . . . and when you get to five . . . all done! Five hops . . . and done! Have fun practicing!*

With older children and teens, I provide the recording of the actual session for them to listen to and may do a brief recording like the one above simply to provide practice in a simple, accessible way. Heavy Hands is another tool that kids can use to develop confidence in their skills in a general way, first using a personalized recording, and then doing it on their own in a variety of settings.

For those children who are ready and willing to independently use their skills (and that is the goal), Gardner (1981) offered a process that teaches the child how to independently move in and out of a hypnotic state. I've summarized it here:

1. First go through a few inductions, choosing ones that a child could use on her own, for example, an eye fixation or counting backward. (Using the induction of looking at the face on the fingernail that I talked about earlier could work, too.) Allow the child to choose her favorite.

2. Have the child practice the preferred induction with you, with instructions on how to come out of hypnosis, by counting up or taking a few deep breaths. Add the suggestion, "You can come out of hypnosis any time you like, just by deciding to" so that the child will have the ability to end her self-hypnosis immediately if circumstances demand that.

3. Have the child go into hypnosis alone, with you as silent company. Gardner suggested having the child nod as a signal when she is in hypnosis, which you then acknowledge simply. Then have the child realert, again on her own.

4. After a few practices, have the parents observe the process, and include questions and answers between the parent and child during the session, so that the parents and child can experience communicating while in hypnosis.

Homework Assignments

In addition to listening to the recordings and practicing self-hypnosis, children routinely get additional homework assignments that support and make real the suggestions made in our sessions together. Research shows that homework assignments with adults improve therapeutic outcomes (Kazantzis, Deane, & Ronan, 2000; Kazantzis & Lampropoulos, 2002). Research with children is lacking, but cognitive-behavioral therapy (CBT) treatment that includes homework has been shown to be effective, particularly with childhood anxiety (Hudson & Kendall, 2002; Hughes & Kendall, 2007). Because some children do react negatively to the term *homework*, I often call it *practice*. I establish this expectation early by stating, "The sessions here with me will teach you something that you will practice out there in your everyday life." Most children are familiar with the concept that practice matters, but if you need to strengthen this concept, seed it early.

The practice experiences you create should strengthen the associations you have made in the session (Yapko, 2010c) and give children a chance to do something that illustrates and activates the seeds you planted in your hypnotic work (Haley, 1973; Zeig, 1990). What is your goal? Do you want to provide an opportunity for competence? Does a child need to experience a resource in action? Or do you need to shake up a rigid pattern or belief? Sometimes an anxious child needs to experience his discomfort or manage his awkwardness. Sometimes a stubborn teenager needs to learn the value of gathering other perspectives by noticing her own rigidity.

For example, April decided during her junior year that she needed to focus only on the school assignments directly connected to her goal of being a graphic artist. Her high school grades were either A (in her art classes) or F (in everything else). Despite many lectures by her mother about the problems with this approach (no top art school was going to dismiss the many Fs in core subjects), April held firm to her all-or-nothing approach, while refusing to get any accurate information about art school admission policies. "I am not going to do anything I don't like to do," was her mantra. We did a hypnosis session on the dangers of black-and-white thinking. This teenage girl found many "close-minded" political positions abhorrent; therefore, eliciting a reaction against stubborn, ill-informed stances was easy. I used the session to strengthen her own belief in "the value of having an open mind." I then gave her the task of reporting back to me with three historical beliefs that we now know to be ridiculous, even dangerous, and three current positions that irritated her own "accepting" values.

For young children, finding (and reading) a book—with the help of Mom or Dad as needed—that illustrates courage, flexibility, making friends, and so on, is a favorite homework assignment. The goal is to be creative, playful, but specific in your assignments. Both parents and children benefit from the "ah ha!" moments of an enlightening homework experience, and from feelings of accomplishment as they report their out-in-the-world successes.

HANDLING THE UNEXPECTED

I can honestly say that most children and teens find the experience of learning and practicing hypnosis positive, interesting, and productive. Most, but not all. If you work with children, you already know that the best-laid plans and intentions can fall flat. You're already capable of handling the unexpected. Here are some common potential stumbling blocks with hypnosis and approaches to manage them.

- If a child is hesitant to participate in hypnosis: Build rapport by acknowledging his point of view. "I don't blame you at all. . . . Maybe you have questions you want to ask, or ideas you want to share. Maybe part of you is curious about what we're going to do together, but part of you thinks it's a bad idea. Or new. Or strange. Or fun. Let's switch gears and do something else." Children can refuse to do anything, anytime. The more informal your hypnotic process, the less likely they will even know they have something to refuse. Therefore, making your interventions a smooth and inclusive part of your interactions works well. If older children balk at a more formal process, simply shift to a conversational approach. A teen who was interested in using hypnosis opened her eyes a few seconds in and let me know she decided it was "weird" and she didn't like it. We just decided instead to talk about the problem and the solutions. I focused on being hypnotic, so that she didn't have to do hypnosis.

- If a child is angry, or refuses to talk or identify a problem: In a therapeutic setting, children are at times embarrassed or angry when problems are brought up—problems they see as no longer an issue or "already over." Psychotherapy has a reputation for talking about what has happened in the past. Kids aren't thrilled with this negative cataloging—and who can blame them? When kids get angry and refuse to talk about what has happened (or why their parents brought them to see me in the first place), I take the opportunity to lead the child toward a future-oriented, problem-solving stance: "I understand what you mean! Who wants to talk about all that stuff? And more importantly, who wants to go back and do that same thing all over again? You can already remember what you need to change, can't you? So I'm with you. Dump that old stuff if you like—let it go—make room for something new—those old patterns and old stories are getting old. You're growing out of them, like shoes that don't fit you anymore. I say let's move forward!"

- If a child gets worse: Sometimes symptoms get worse, and it would be a mistake to attribute the worsening symptoms to the hypnosis session alone, just as it would be a mistake to attribute improvement of symptoms to hypnosis alone. Hypnosis, as I hope is clear by now, is a way to amplify, create, and discover resources with the goal of improving functioning in some way. Each child, each symptom, and each possible solution must be considered in the same manner that we approach those under our care: commensurate with our training and expertise. From sleep to headaches to anxiety to tics, we must always flexibly evaluate what's working and what's not, and hypnosis can and should be only one of the possible tools considered to remedy a situation.

- Or just doesn't improve: Less dramatic are the situations when the child just stays the same. Bedtime remains problematic; headaches don't lessen; angry explosions occur as frequently. Assuming physical factors have been addressed when indicated, now is the time to consider interrupting your own patterns. What can you do differently? Are you aiming for the right target? Can you focus on the response set in order to build more momentum toward the frame you wish to amplify? Are you being too indirect? Too direct? How might you be more curious and collaborative as you work together with the child? What might you address in the family context? After all, client sessions are periodic, compared to the ongoing reinforcement of patterns at home.

You now have the ingredients and the general recipe to create targeted and individualized sessions. You've learned how to use the first session to build rapport and set a hopeful and expectant tone. You know to match your style and energy to the developmental needs of the child. You understand the importance of identifying the right target, building momentum toward the goal of a new and improved frame. You can imagine an absorbing and playful experience that shows a child a new pattern, a different path. The next chapters will help you take what you've learned and apply it to childhood struggles and challenges, knowing, of course, that the connection and creativity between you and the child are the keys to doing this well.

CHAPTER *6*

Hypnosis and Anxiety

Stepping in,
Moving Forward

*A*nxiety has done well for itself. By all accounts it is one of the most prevalent mental health disorders in children, with lifetime prevalence of "any anxiety disorder" in children or adolescents about 15% to 20% (Beesdo, Knappe, & Pine, 2009). Separation anxiety and specific phobias show up first, with social anxiety and panic disorder arriving later, often emerging with adolescence. When left untreated, anxiety has staying power, causing impairment in a child's social and academic functioning that remains constant through the teen years and into adulthood (Beesdo et al., 2009). Anxiety also likes company. Anxiety disorders in childhood are predictors of multiple other psychiatric disorders in adolescence (Bittner et al., 2007; Wagner, 2005), particularly depression and substance abuse. The most common comorbid pattern by far is that of anxiety and depressive disorders, with anxiety frequently showing up first. One analysis found that among those with both anxiety and depression, 72% had anxiety first (Essau, 2003). Peer connection is often impacted: the coping strategies of the anxious child (namely withdrawal and avoidance) often lead to isolation, thus preventing him from learning important social skills and developing helpful peer support that encourages positive risk taking and courage (Hudson, Flannery-Schroeder, & Kendall, 2004).

What causes anxiety? The answer, not surprisingly, appears to be a combination of genes, family influences, and other environmental factors. Temperament, particularly behavioral inhibition, has been long identified as a risk factor (Kagan, Reznick, Clarke, Snidman, & Garcia-Coll, 1984; Kagan, Reznick, & Snidman, 1987). Parenting style, insecure attachment (Esbjorn, Bender, Reinholdt-Dunne, Munck, & Ollendick, 2012), and maternal depression and anxiety also come into play (McLeod, Wood, & Weisz, 2007). Research suggests that a parent's perception of the world's dangers and the expression of these fears add to a child's anxiety (Bagner et al., 2013; Creswell & O'Connor, 2006). Drake & Ginsburg (2012b) found it difficult to synthesize all the research on parents and their anxious children, concluding that, despite clear correlations, causality and directionality are still up for debate. Trauma and stressful life events can obviously lead to anxiety, although how a child and her caretakers perceive and manage these events may modulate the anxious response (Rapee et al., 1990).

Whatever the source, a certain cognitive frame is central to the development and maintenance of anxiety: a perceived lack of control over external threats, combined with a lack of control over one's internal emotional and bodily reactions (Barlow, 2001; Weems, Silverman, Rapee, & Pina, 2003). In other words, an anxious child perceives his world as a scary place (sometimes this is an accurate assessment, sometimes not), and his emotions and body react strongly to the potential dangers.

The good news is that intervention for anxiety works (e.g., Piacentini et al., 2014; Wood, Piacentini, Southam-Gerow, Chu, & Sigman, 2006; Schneider et al., 2011). When children and their parents learn how anxiety operates, and then are taught how to handle its predictable maneuvers, they improve significantly. Promising programs with behaviorally inhibited children and their parents show that brief and early intervention matters (McLoone, Hudson, & Rapee, 2006; Rapee, Kennedy, Ingram, Edwards, & Sweeney, 2005; Teubert & Pinquart, 2011). A brief group program for at-risk families (defined as anxious parents and their as-yet not anxious children) focused on psychoeducation, problem solving, tolerance of uncertainty, and parenting skills. A year later, 30% of the control group children were identified as anxious, while 0% of the children in the treatment group had developed symptoms (Ginsburg, 2009). And if you ask clinicians (like me) who work with anxious kids and families, we'll tell you that successful treatment is commonplace.

Anxious children step back from life, desperate to avoid feeling overwhelmed, incompetent, or scared. And avoidance works. When they step away from their fear, they feel better. Simple as that. But when they avoid, they miss out—not only on positive events and successes, but on the experiences of failing and recovering, the triumph of not knowing at first but figuring it out eventually, and the feeling of mastery based on experiential learning. Therefore, to effectively use hypnosis with anxious children, the hypnotic interventions, self-hypnosis, and homework assignments must point the child in a different direction. We must suggest, inspire, and elicit responses and skills that are the opposite of what anxiety demands in its bossy, repetitive way.

Reid Wilson and I outlined our approach to helping children and parents decrease anxiety in our book *Anxious Kids, Anxious Parents: 7 Ways to Stop the Worry Cycle and Raise Courageous and Independent Children* (Wilson & Lyons, 2013), which is based on a few key principles:

1. Anxiety is a natural, expected process that sometimes serves a purpose. The content of worry (the triggers) may change, but the process remains the same. When children learn about the process of anxiety—which is predictable and redundant—rather than focusing on the content of the worry, they can develop umbrella skills that move with them through the life cycle and anxiety's many manifestations.

2. Because worry and the resultant anxiety demand certainty and comfort, equipping a child with internal resources to (a) tolerate the inevitable uncertainty and discomfort of her external world and (b) create new responses is essential.

3. Working to get rid of anxiety—which is understandably what all children and parents want to do—actually makes anxiety stronger. Therefore, interventions that promote calmness and escape (such as relaxation or going to a safe place) must be seen as only part of an overall strategy that supports and induces a bigger shift in responding and reacting. Strategies should not enhance an anxious child's natural tendency to suppress, distract, or avoid (Barlow, Allen, & Choate, 2004; Amstadter, 2008; Hofman, Heering, Sawyer, & Asnaani, 2009). As Amstadter concluded, "Suppression, while theoretically employed in efforts to decrease emotional experiencing, appears to paradoxically increase symptoms of anxiety and distress" (2008, p. 216).

Let's take the three frames described in Chapter 4 and the sequential components of Chapter 5, combine them with what we know about effective anxiety treatment, and create successful interventions. In the next section, I take each of the frames and give examples for possible inductions, response sets, and suggestions that give kids broad and usable skills. Remember, anxiety wraps itself around many different contents and diagnoses, but its process is consistent.

Note: Whenever I give a series of examples, I'll start with

younger children and progress to older children and more complex examples. That way, I won't have to repeatedly distinguish the intended age group or developmental level, which would get tedious for us both.

- Experience is variable (vs. rigid and permanent)
- The value of parts (vs. global and overwhelming)
  - Sequencing
  - Compartmentalizing
  - Connection and disconnection, or signals and noise
- Action counts (vs. passive and avoidant)

EXPERIENCE IS VARIABLE: LET'S GET UNCERTAIN

As I said in Chapter 4, the idea of variability and flexibility is useful in practically every encounter with a child, but when addressing the rigidity of anxiety, this theme moves to the front of the line. Why? Because anxiety is a one-trick pony that gains power by demanding a rigid response. While it has learned to look and feel overwhelming and complicated, its rules are simple: "I have to know how this will go!" (certainty) and "I have to feel okay! I have to calm down!" (comfort). Anxiety convinces children (and adults) of their inadequacy by predictably announcing, "You can't handle this!" And its options for relief are narrow: "Avoid this now or things will get really bad!"

Unfortunately, hypnosis with anxious children has historically relied almost exclusively on suggestions and techniques that focus on the creation of relaxation and calmness. Why do I say "unfortunately"? Because what anxious kids really need is an increased ability to tolerate uncertainty and actively problem solve. If techniques of breathing, relaxation, and elimination of worry are the primary hypnotic interventions, this has the potential to feed into anxiety's unrealistic and rigid demands for comfort. This then validates the anxious child's quest to "get rid of worry" (Wilson & Lyons, 2013).

Breathing exercises in the treatment of panic have long been seen as avoidant safety behaviors (Clark, 1986), meaning that they are used to avoid or escape anxious thoughts and sensations, hindering the development of new responses. Suggestions for comfort and relaxation ("All your worries can just float away" or "You can imagine feeling completely calm and relaxed as you try out for the team") make the elimination of uncertainty or stressful events a necessary precursor to moving toward the feared stimulus. This is the very agenda that stops an anxious child in his tracks (Wilson & Lyons, 2013).

What can we do instead? Use hypnosis to help normalize and adjust to emotional and physical arousal. When kids learn to expect and reframe anxiety's predictable arrival—rather than focus on eliminating it—they do better. Research with test-taking teens and socially anxious adults supports the notion that performance improves when anxiety symptoms and arousal are interpreted differently, creating significant positive effects on emotions, physiology, and behavior (Jamieson, Mendes, Blackstock, & Schmader, 2010; Beltzer, Nock, Peters, & Jamieson, 2014).

Breathing and relaxation exercises can fit into this approach wonderfully when they are introduced as a way to "reboot" before moving forward. Rather than seeing breathing exercises as a way to calm down, relax, and eliminate anxiety (which is how they are frequently presented), they can be introduced as one part of a broader strategy that teaches anxious children how to handle physical and emotional arousal. For example, a child can learn to take three calming breaths as she allows herself to notice her anxiety talking: "I can hear what my anxiety is saying . . . and my calming breaths remind me that I can handle my brain and my body. . . . Three breaths give me a chance to focus on how I'm learning and changing." Simply stated, anxious children can and must learn more than how to relax, for not only is this often an unrealistic goal (we all feel worry and anxiety), it hinders the development of the important skills of tolerating uncertainty, discriminating between helpful and unhelpful thoughts, and stepping into challenges (Wilson & Lyons, 2013).

Keep in mind that children with physical symptoms and comorbid conditions that are exacerbated by anxiety (such as asthma or headaches) will benefit more from an early focus on relaxation techniques for two important reasons: (1) they'll experience a decrease in the physical symptoms that are interfering with functioning, allowing for more anxiety-related work to be done; and (2) they will begin to understand the connection between emotional reactions and physical symptoms and their ability to impact this. (I discuss the use of hypnosis with physical symptoms in Chapter 8.)

Hypnosis is a great tool to help a child reappraise and adjust her thoughts and reactions to anxiety's rules. An effective session destabilizes anxiety's rigid pattern and demonstrates how responses to thoughts and physical sensations can be altered (Kaiser, 2014; Golden 2012). I encourage you to focus your interventions on developing an anxious child's ability to "not know" and be okay, to feel "uncomfortable" and step forward anyway. Remember the goal: managing the variability of internal and external experiences and a tolerance of uncertainty that ultimately give a child more autonomy.

Induction

The induction itself is an invitation to

- Try something new
- Play a new game
- Do something cool
- Listen to a story
- Help me tell a story
- Use your imagination in a fun way
- Experience yourself in a different way

• Take some time to focus on new ways of responding to old messages

However you choose to introduce this change of focus or new experience is fine. Remember, it's simply a brief way of orienting and focusing the child's attention. Of course, seeding flexibility, newness, change, and malleability paves the way for what's to come, so drop a few hints.

For more extended inductions, you may choose to create a physical experience of variability. All the ideas presented in Chapter 5 can be used and adapted to introduce the broader concept of malleability illustrated by changing one's physical state in some way. Heavy Hands, for example, can be offered in a shortened version as an example of how "you create a feeling in your body just by thinking about it." Playing around with making one hand heavy while another feels "as usual" or even lighter than usual is a fun way to show a child how powerful the imagination can be, and how it connects to responses in the body.

Building a Response Set Toward Variability and Malleability

When targeting the rigidity of anxiety, the response set continues to lead the child in the direction of variability and malleability. Truisms about how we can feel one way on one day and another way the next, how different people have different tastes and opinions, or how we change from moment to moment all connect to the desired new frame: life is variable, on the inside and the outside, and flexibility is required. Changing, shifting, adapting—all of these suggest an alternative frame to anxiety's rigidity. Look to include general statements about physical variability, too, because anxious children want comfort and often respond strongly (and with alarm) to any physical (albeit normal) symptoms of anxiety, a pattern referred to as anxiety sensitivity (Silverman, Fleisig, Rabian, & Peterson, 1991).

In Chapter 5, I described a possible response set with a girl frightened by new experiences. (There's that need for certainty.) The response set was full of truisms about how things change—things we can control and things we can't. Here are some additional examples:

> Some kids go to bed at 7 and others have a later bedtime . . .
> and some kids love cats and others love dogs and some love all
> different kinds of animals . . . and some kids love to take baths
> and other kids fight to stay dirty. . . . Kids are so different . . .
> and they change all the time! It might be hard to count all the
> ways that you have changed since you were a little kid. . . .

> Experts might say you need 8 hours of sleep, but some people
> prefer 7 and some prefer 10. . . . And the feeling you get on a
> roller-coaster ride is fun for one kid and awful for another. . . .
> And you might enjoy a surprise party when you're 9, but hate it
> when you're 16 . . . or really not mind either way. . . .

> Sometimes you crave ice cream and other times you want pret-
> zels. . . . And sometimes you feel like you'll ace a test and
> other times you're less sure. . . . Sometimes we're certain it's
> going to rain, and it does . . . but sometimes that rainy forecast
> becomes a surprisingly sunny day. . . .

The "I don't know" set is a great way to promote uncertainty:

> I don't know exactly how you've changed since you were little,
> or how tall you'll end up being . . . or what color your first car
> will be . . . or even when you'll learn to drive . . . and maybe
> you don't either. . . . How could you, really? . . . With so much

still ahead of you. . . .

Erickson introduced the use of hypnosis itself as a way to courageously step into new territory (Erickson et al., 1976). I think it's a great suggestion to anxious teens as it portends what they'll eventually need to do outside of the therapeutic experience as well:

> *And one of the nicest things about hypnosis is that in the trance*
> *state you can dare to look at and think and see and feel things*
> *that you wouldn't dare in the ordinary waking state. . . . (p. 35)*

In sum, you want to suggest—in broad, nonthreatening, and indisputable ways—that life is a changing and unpredictable experience, both internally and externally.

You're now ready to move into your suggestions—and I say this knowing you've already made lots of suggestions—with this question in mind: How will I help this anxious child further develop the ability to be malleable in the face of life's uncertainties, the opposite of what anxiety demands?

The Intervention and Suggestions

I find it helpful to distill the message I plan to convey into a sentence or two. Here are a few examples:

1. Anxiety is rigid, but you can create flexible responses in your body and your thoughts.
2. Handling uncertainty is a part of life . . . and you are learning to handle it.
3. Now you know anxiety's game . . . so let's expect it to show up and do its same old thing. No more surprises, no more playing by anxiety's rules.

Once you have the message, you can use a combination of stories, direct suggestions, rehearsal imagery, or role-playing. This is where your flexibility comes into play.

The following are some examples of suggestions for the three options above (remember: youngest to oldest) including a check-in and posthypnotic suggestion for each.

Anxiety Is Rigid, but You Can Be Flexible

We've talked about how bossy your worry can be . . . how it makes so many rules . . . and when worry is in charge . . . it makes you just like a piece of uncooked spaghetti. . . . Can you imagine an uncooked piece of spaghetti? [I suggest having some dry spaghetti on hand.] . . . You can't bend it or twist it, or it will break. . . . Just like worry wants you to be so careful. . . . It wants you to be stiff . . . with all your muscles tight. . . . Can you do that right now? Make all your muscles as tight as can be . . . your arms, your legs, your spine. [Model this posture.] . . . How uncomfortable! It makes it hard to do much at all . . . but a cooked piece of spaghetti is wiggly and loose and flexible. . . . You can bend it and make it into a circle or a letter S. . . . Can you be a piece of wiggly loose spaghetti right now? Can you let your arms and legs and face be so loose? . . . Worry has been making the rules . . . telling you what you can and can't do . . . making you think that you're as delicate as that uncooked spaghetti . . . but you can be loose and run and play and ride your bike with all your energy . . . and go on new adventures and try different things. . . . Oh, that worry will show up. . . . It thinks it's the boss . . . telling you how to be stiff and stubborn. . . . Now you have something else to do. . . . Let's do it again together. . . .

Throughout the session, it's likely that you've been checking in and conversing, particularly with younger children. Validate what the child shares (or if he's confused or not understanding, it's important to clarify) and then reiterate your message simply and directly.

This moves you right into the posthypnotic suggestion, especially with younger children. (It's a very fluid process.) As described in Chapter 5, the goal here is to connect what you have just done together to the child's experiences in her world:

When you're in situation XX, you'll be able to do YY.

Worry wants you to be stiff and fragile like this piece of spaghetti. But you can show worry how to be loose and flexible, with your body and your mind, can't you? When worry shows up again . . . do you know when that will happen? Any ideas? . . . When it happens, you can remember how to be a flexible cooked piece of spaghetti. . . . Can you show me now? Great! And you can listen to this whenever you like . . . to remind you of how you can break worry's rules. . . .

Handling Uncertainty; Responding Differently to Anxiety

And I've been talking to you about how different people learn to handle different things . . . and how things that were hard when we're little seem so automatic as we grow. . . . And I wonder how long your list might be. . . . If you think for a minute about first grade and second grade all the way to fifth grade . . . all the new things you did that are hardly new anymore . . . and the times you felt awkward or scared or nervous. . . . When you first went up to bat this season . . . or presented your project to your class . . . or even the first time you came to my office . . . of course you couldn't know exactly what would happen . . . but we know that worry has one message. . . . Over and over it's told you to

148

stop. . . . It says you have to know! . . . It's told your brain to tell your body to [fill in physical symptoms] . . . and sometimes you listened to worry. . . . You didn't know what worry was up to . . . When I was a kid, I listened, too . . . until I learned that I had a choice . . . to be bored or annoyed instead. . . . Isn't that interesting? . . . And there's a story about another boy you might like to hear. . . . This boy named Evan told me about his next-door neighbor . . . a neighbor boy named Ted . . . who always gave bad advice. . . . Ted told Evan to do things . . . and Evan learned not to listen to Ted. . . . He knew Ted would show up . . . and he didn't really mind . . . especially after he learned to let Ted's advice go in one ear and out the other. . . . And when I asked Evan to name his worry . . . his predictable, boring worry . . . you can guess what name he chose. . . . He already had lots of practice handling Ted . . . and this brought a smile to his face . . . which is a nice thing to do in the face of worry. . . .

Check in as needed:

Have you been thinking about the many things you've learned as you've grown? . . . And now how you're learning to handle worry, too? Is there anything you'd like to share with me about what you can handle or what you've learned?

Offer the posthypnotic suggestion:

So the next time your worry shows up, like Ted coming over to Evan's house, I wonder how it will go. . . . Will it go in one ear and out the other? Or will it visit your brain or your tummy? Wherever it shows up, you can remember our time together . . . and when you listen to this recording . . . you can practice in your imagination . . . and I can't wait to hear how your worry will try to give you bad advice . . . and maybe you'll show me . . . unless you'd like to show me right now. . . . [Look for opportunities with kids to do some role-playing to seal the deal.]

Let's Expect Anxiety and Change the Rules

I ran into an old high school friend the other day. . . . I hadn't seen him in 30 years. . . . He was quiet and kind in high school. . . . He told me that he was a lawyer now . . . and after law school he went into trial law . . . which meant he had to stand up in front of a judge and jury and make his case . . . and there was often a lot on the line. . . . So he told himself to stay calm . . . *to stop worrying about the mistakes he might make . . . but then he'd remind himself that* mistakes weren't allowed. . . . *You can't make mistakes when the stakes are so high . . . so as he talked to the jury, his worry would show up . . . and his left leg would begin to shake . . . and when he tried to stop it . . . it only got worse. . . . And he wondered how his clients felt . . . seeing the shaking . . . and how the judge must have judged him right there . . . until, he told me, he read an interview with a famous rock star . . . Sting from the Police . . . and Sting said he would get nervous before a show . . . and he tried everything to stop it . . . to relax his body . . . until he decided he was* supposed *to feel that way . . . because he wanted to perform well . . . and his body and brain were getting ready. . . . And he couldn't know exactly what would happen out there . . . so* of course *he felt nervous. . . . It meant he cared. . . . And my friend the lawyer decided that he was like a rock star who wanted to do well . . . to step onto the stage . . . and his shaky leg was just a reminder that this was important . . . and he stopped stopping it . . . just let it be there . . . and he thanked his leg for the message . . . which confused his worry . . . which was fine with him. . . . And the funny thing is . . . when he stopped stopping his leg . . . stopped working so hard on stopping it . . . it slowed way down . . . on its own . . . to a little shake. . . .*

Check in:

> *I've been doing the talking for a while, and I'm curious to know what you've been thinking about as I've been talking. . . . Will you share your thoughts with me? Any ideas or reactions to what I've said?*

Utilize what's offered and reiterate the therapeutic message:

> *Yes, you're really understanding. . . . It's important to know you have options . . . that you can feel unsure and handle it . . . and that worry and anxiety show up, a normal part of growing and learning . . . and you can recognize it . . . even expect it. . . . That's a different way of responding . . . which can sometimes mean not needing to respond at all . . . which you can practice. . . .*

Offer a posthypnotic suggestion:

> *And you can look for times to practice . . . for chances to show yourself what you're capable of . . . to step into situations that you care about, that have meaning, and that might even be challenging, . . . and to know what's happening . . . and to think about it in a different way . . . to notice how your mind and body can welcome new habits and reactions . . . and even the noticing itself is the start of a new habit . . . isn't it?*

THE VALUE OF PARTS: SEQUENCING, COMPARTMENTALIZING, DISCRIMINATING

We now move on to the importance of parts, which builds upon the flexibility work above. The concept of parts when dealing with anxiety is important because it vividly counteracts the common cognitive errors of anxious kids: overgeneralization or global thinking, cata-strophizing, personalizing, and selective abstraction, a focus on the negative aspects of an experience (Leitenberg, Yost, & Carroll-Wilson, 1986; Weems et al., 2001). Anxious kids who get overwhelmed and then seek to avoid must develop the ability to break down an experience into manageable chunks, get a bit of distance from their own anxiety, and sort through what's important and what's not. These skills are the antidote to the all-or-nothing approach of anxious kids. Because these cognitive patterns are also present in depressed children, and the link between childhood anxiety and the development of depression is well established (Beesdo et al., 2009; Weems et al., 2001), these skills also serve an important preventative role in what often become chronic and comorbid disorders.

Sequencing: One Step at a Time

Remember Bethany, the college-bound high school senior in Chapter 4, who paralyzed herself with thoughts of all that she had to accomplish? Anxious children leap far into the future, imagining how they will handle that big life challenge ahead, without much consideration for how many steps (and opportunities to learn) they will have along the way.

Your job in the hypnosis session is to introduce sequencing and steps as a normal, helpful, and inevitable part of growing and learning. Illustrate a different relationship between the present and the future, as it is this projection into the unknown and oft-perceived catastrophic future that fuels the worrier's cry, "I can't handle this!"

Induction

Use your induction to introduce a sequence, which is a common and popular approach used in many situations, even when sequencing is not the specific frame or skill being introduced.

First, let's get comfortable. . . . Let's shift our bodies and find an easy way to sit . . . and then we can take a nice breath together, just to settle in a bit . . . and step by step you can let your hands get heavier, and then your feet, and then your eyelids . . . and slowly but steadily . . . you focus a bit more on focusing a bit more. . . .

Any variation of a step-by-step progression is fine, for example, going down a staircase, or simply counting down from 10 to 1, or relaxing from head to toe.

Building a Response Set Toward Steps and Sequences

The response set continues along the theme of steps—their importance, their helpfulness, and their role in so much of what we do. The suggestions then expand upon the theme of steps and how they move us into the future, gathering experience and knowledge as we go.

So as we sit here together, taking breaths together . . . it's nice not to rush . . . sometimes to just notice the steps we take . . . the steps from busy to still . . . or how we go from playing to listening. . . . Many big things are full of little steps . . . like building a house . . . or planting a garden . . . all the steps a bear takes to get ready to hibernate for the winter . . . or how the robin builds her nest in the spring . . . one twig at a time . . . one piece of grass. . . .

Or:

Many things have a beginning and an end . . . recipes . . . math problems . . . and the alphabet . . . and musical notes like do re mi . . . and when we're figuring things out . . . trying

something new or learning the ropes . . . those steps . . . those
directions . . . can help us move ahead step by step. . . . We
learn our letters . . . and then the sounds of the letters . . . and
then how to put them together in words . . . and sentences . . .
and paragraphs. . . .

Interventions and Suggestions

The goal of the intervention is to help the child internalize a different way (based on steps and sequences) of assessing and then approaching an experience. Metaphors that build on the language of steps, taking things in order, and appreciating the time it takes to go from beginner to expert are all helpful.

Henry, for example, was an 8-year-old with separation anxiety and a not-so-helpful imagination (at least not in the way he was employing it of late). Whenever anyone in his family talked about "going away," for example, to summer camp, on a vacation, on a business trip, or to college (he had a brother in high school), Henry would cry and yell, demanding that they stop talking. He told me when we met that when he heard others talk about going away, he imagined what it would be like when he had to go away, something he had never done. I told Henry he had a lot to learn about his worry, but we could start with his Jump Ahead problem, his habit of jumping ahead to something big and scary in his imagination, without spending any time imagining and practicing how he'd learn to handle what 8-year-olds are supposed to handle, based on the fact that they are 8.

Henry loved to build with Legos, so I said:

L: You know, I've seen those big Lego sets . . . the ones with thousands of pieces. . . . The instruction book is this thick. . . . Do you remember your first Lego set? Was it something simple?

HENRY: Yes, I had a little fire engine.

L: It would probably be boring to you now. . . .

HENRY: I don't play with it anymore.

L: And the last one you got for your birthday . . . the one you told me about . . . that took you how many hours to build?

HENRY: Eight hours! It was hard!

L: Can you imagine right now, with that great imagination of yours, what that pile of Legos looked like, dumped out on the floor . . . before you even put one piece together? You couldn't have done that when you were 5 . . . no way. . . . But now you know how to follow the directions . . . how to move from one step to the next . . . and you can imagine getting an even bigger set . . . the one that costs so much money you'll have to start saving up now . . . and you won't even have it for years probably. . . .

HENRY: I am saving now. I think I will get it when I'm 10.

L: I think we can learn something about your worry . . . your Jumping Ahead habit, if we think about Legos. . . . With Legos you build and learn and get better as you go . . . but your worry doesn't let you learn. . . . Your worry makes you think and imagine, but it doesn't let you *do stuff and learn stuff step by step*. . . . Your worry thinks about Jason going to college . . . and imagines *you* going to college . . . without even letting you learn first. . . . And what worry doesn't know . . . is that we're going to start imagining how to handle him. . . . You can learn about worry. . . . He's like that little Lego set that has become boring . . . not so complicated at all. . . . And step by step you're going to outgrow him, too . . . boring as he is . . . and then you'll start learning *how to visit places* and *handle new things*. . . .

HENRY: Maybe I'll build a Lego worry guy and bring him to you.

Posthypnotic Suggestion

I love that idea! And while you're building that worry guy, I want you to think about how much you know about building with Legos. You won't even need any directions to build that guy. . . . You have so much experience. . . . And when you hear someone talking about going somewhere, going away, you can think about Legos and remember that you're learning how to handle that, too. There are some steps to take first. . . . You will learn about worry and what it does . . . and learn what to say when worry gets in the way of you doing and building and growing. . . . I'm so glad you are a builder of things. . . . Builders know how to take it a step at a time. . . . Even if they jump ahead and imagine . . . they still have to back up and build it. . . .

Too Much of a Good Thing

Before we move ahead, there's one caveat to consider when it comes to sequencing and anxious kids: sometimes, a rigid dependence on steps and sequencing (by the child, parent, and even the therapist) is the problem. The solution then lies in the ability to determine when to follow the steps and when to be more flexible. Anxious children want certainty; therefore they may become excessively reliant on planning and knowing exactly what's going to happen, demanding that parents and other adults provide and follow detailed steps and routines. Consider the perfectionist who is so worried about making an error or forgetting something that she packs and repacks her backpack multiple times before going to bed at night. In such cases, sequencing can be taught as an independent skill done by the child in the face of a large or overwhelming task, but you must also introduce an appreciation for flexibility. The message thus becomes: "Sometimes steps are helpful and important, but sometimes—once we know what we're doing—we can shake it up a bit or skip some steps . . . and you are learning to tell the difference."

Leora Kuttner (2009) illustrated this movement away from sequence as she described the use of hypnosis with an 11-year-old anxious girl with long-standing sleep difficulties. The girl and her mother were locked into a dysfunctional bedtime sequence, which wasn't helped by a standard sequential CBT intervention. Using the girl's own hobby of baking cakes, Kuttner used word play, metaphor, and surprise, creating a hypnotic moment that disrupted the rigid sequence. Kuttner concluded, "It has been my experience that the more standard therapeutic protocols with step-by-step approximations to a desired goal, tend to drag out the therapeutic process making the resolution of the anxiety more difficult for highly anxious children" (2009, p. 63). This is important for anxiety and for other issues, too, like depression or pain management: you as therapist can go too slowly, too methodically for the child in front of you. A major value of hypnotic technique, let us not forget, is its ability to speed along the process, which enables the child client to see real progress and experience hope and accomplishment.

Compartmentalization: Breaking It Down

When it comes to managing anxiety, the general umbrella skill of compartmentalization is a game changer. I often tell families that anxiety is like a cult leader that moves in with a family and takes over, overwhelming the family with its rules and demands. The ability to compartmentalize helps a child and family get some distance from anxiety, not as a way to deny its existence or block it out, but as a way to step back from its global overwhelming voice and scary dramatic symptoms. Teaching this skill, especially with younger children, tends to be an active process, with role-playing, props, and art.

When teaching the concept of compartmentalizing, your job is to show an anxious child how to:

1. Externalize the anxiety by giving it a name, drawing a picture of it, and taking it out of our brains and chatting with it
2. Break down global thinking and overwhelming events into more specific categories (similar to the sequencing described above), which helps with the common patterns of overgeneralization and selective abstraction (Weems et al., 2001)
3. Identify the different parts that we all have, parts that make anxiety bigger and parts that help us handle our worries, including the different parts of our brain (the prefrontal cortex, the amygdala) and body (see Yapko's parts metaphor in Hammond, 1990, p. 321)

Here are some brief examples of each.

Helping a 6-Year-Old Externalize Worry

I don't know if you know this, but we all have a worry part, a part inside us that wants to protect us, and make sure that everything goes smoothly. Worry parts can be big or small, bossy or quiet. I'd like to take yours out for a minute and have a look. Would that be okay? It's quite simple. [Pretend to reach over and grab something out of the child's body, and then plop it down in front of you both.] Let's sit here together and have a look. . . . What do you see? [Prompt as needed.] . . . How big is it? Can you show me with your hands? Does it have a color? Some kids like to draw a picture of their worry part and give it a name. You can if you like. . . . Remember what I told you about worry parts? They like to know everything . . . and they tell kids, "Hey, you can't handle that!" So predictable! I wonder if we can talk to your worry part.

. . . What do you think it should know about you?

Spend time getting to know the worry part, allowing the child to be the worry part while you talk back, then switching roles. Continue to emphasize its predictability to counter the alarm response it usually generates. Allow the child to build the worry part, and how to talk to it. Many portray theirs as an evil villain with which to do battle, but I also had a young girl who called her worry "Mouse" and treated it with care and empathy. Both ways work. Which way depends on the incoming temperament of the child in front of you.

After playing, drawing, and so on, focus the child's attention and offer the posthypnotic suggestion:

> *Now that you know your Fred the Worry Part so well, I bet you will know when he shows up next time. You told me he likes to be bossy before school and when you're waiting for the bus, so now you won't be surprised when he shows up and says the same old thing. Do you remember how we talked to Fred? He wants you to be scared, but we giggled a lot, didn't we? So when you're getting ready for school, wait for Fred, and let him know that you know what he's up to. . . . You know how he makes your heart beat faster and your tummy do a flip. Let's practice one more time what you'll say to Fred. . . .*

Helping a 12-Year-Old Break Down Her Pattern of Anticipatory and Global Homework Meltdowns

Following a brief induction, the response set offers truisms about how some things that come easy to one person are harder for someone else, like telling a joke, or reading a map, or whistling, and how some parts of an experience are more enjoyable than others, like going uphill versus downhill on a bike ride, or snuggling a new kitten versus cleaning out the litter box.

And when it comes to school and learning, I bet there are parts that come easy . . . parts that are fun. . . . You told me you are a good speller . . . and I know from looking at the cover of your notebooks that you're a very skilled artist . . . such detail. . . . And some kids love finding the right answer in math . . . while others love the freedom of writing a story . . . but even the math whiz might dread geometry . . . and even the writer might hate proofreading. . . . Most experiences have some good parts and some lousy parts . . . and some people dive into the fun part first . . . but other people save the best for last. . . . But what happens when you decide ahead of time that there is no good, no easy, no quick? . . . That it's all too hard, too boring, too miserable? . . . What do you miss . . . ?

I wonder what it would be like . . . just an experiment . . . to find what works for you . . . knowing of course that there will be some fun and some yuck . . . some uphill, some downhill . . . knowing you probably know the difference. . . . But what will you do first? The dessert or the vegetables? The up or the down? When you sit down to do your homework tomorrow and the next day and the next day . . . what will you do with the easy parts and the tricky parts? How will you create your own plan to play with your homework? . . . And will all of it really be work? . . .

Helping a Shy Teen Identify and Focus on the Parts Needed for a Job Interview

A brief induction invites him to focus on one part at a time and to notice the differences, and to notice that some parts might be more focused and other parts less focused. This moves into a response set that introduces the universal experience of changing one's behavior based on the situation—how kids learn to have an inside voice and an outside voice, and people have a professional voice and a casual voice, especially radio broadcasters and Broadway performers, and how we talk differently with our closest friends compared to our teachers or grandparents.

And we all have different parts of us . . . parts that we show other people and parts that we keep to ourselves . . . a fun part . . . a childish part . . . parts we like and parts we don't. . . . And I remember watching a tennis match with the top player in the world . . . John McEnroe . . . who was known at times to explode. . . . And the announcer said . . . "I wonder which McEnroe will show up today." . . . And Don Rickles was a loud comedian who said in an interview, "I'm very shy, so I became outgoing so I could protect my shyness." . . . And Johnny Depp has said he never wanted to be famous, but then became a movie star. . . . And of course we know that we're made up of many parts . . . but it's interesting to think about what part is bigger and louder. . . . You can have that one part that wants a job . . . and several parts that know you can do the job . . . and want the money . . . and another part, that quiet part, that worries about what you'll say. . . . And while most of you can be ready to take the risk . . . you can let that quiet part be there loudly if it wants . . . but you don't have to listen. . . . While you focus on what you want . . . the parts of having a job that matter to you . . . you can imagine that part . . . that shy part . . . how it shows up . . . makes your face red . . . or makes your heart pound . . . and like Don Rickles . . . you can have that part . . . and you can imagine right now . . . talking in the interview . . . even with your shyness checking in . . . there's no surprise. . . . It's nothing new . . . and you can put it somewhere inside of you . . . or outside of you. . . . You can know it's there . . . and just let it be there and do its job . . . while you get yours. . . .

And then the posthypnotic suggestion:

And whenever you listen to this over the next few days . . . practicing how you'll notice your shy part . . . maybe rehearsing in your mind walking into the interview . . . all of you . . . feeling the nervous feelings . . . feelings that aren't new . . . and focusing on the job at hand . . . shaking hands . . . saying hello . . . heart pounding on the inside, of course, as expected . . . because you want this . . . and knowing that just one part is worried. . . . But you have so many other parts of you to answer and listen and do the work. . . . That's a good feeling to have . . . and after a while, you just might forget about that shy part because there will no longer be something to be shy about. . . .

Signals Versus Noise: When to Listen, When to Ignore

This last skill goes after anxiety's inability to differentiate between what's important and what's not. Anxious children have a hard time determining what to ignore and what to amplify. They are connected to their worried thoughts, their somatic symptoms, and to the perceived threats around them, but are often impervious to the positives that surround them, including their successes, strengths, and enjoyable experiences (Taghavi, Dalgleish, Moradi, Neshat-Doost, & Yule, 2003; Dadds, Barrett, Rapee, & Ryan, 1996; Bogels & Zigterman, 2000; Weems et al., 2001).

If we follow the basic tenet of hypnosis that "what you focus on you amplify," anxious children, because of their cognitive and attentional biases toward threat and negativity, are attending to their worries about the negatives that might happen, and minimizing their focus on what they can handle (Esbjorn et al., 2012). We also know that anxious parents and children interpret ambiguous stimuli as more dangerous (Creswell & O'Connor, 2006). All in all, it's safe to say that anxious children—and often their parents—have a tendency to seek out the thundercloud lurking behind every silver lining.

This skill is closely related to externalizing, as the goal is to put some distance between the child and her anxious thoughts, while also allowing for the retrieval and amplification of positive experiences. The message here is "Just because you think it doesn't make it so" (Michael Yapko, personal communication, 2005). For many anxious kids, the message must also be "Just because you heard about it doesn't mean it's going to happen to you." Without a filter for one's internal imaginings or the news of the world, life is scary and overwhelming. Without the ability to sort through the negatives and discover the positives, it's pretty depressing, too.

I remember meeting with a 10-year-old girl and her mother. Although I certainly appreciate when someone hangs on my every word, this girl's vigilant, almost unblinking attention became a bit unnerving. Because she was so worried about potential dangers in her world, she constantly monitored adults for signs of alarm or possible dangers. When I made the mistake of mentioning another client who had successfully dealt with a similar fear (not hers), her eyes grew even bigger as she cried, "Now you've given my brain something else to worry about! What if I get that fear?"

As you create interventions that focus on the ability to discriminate and filter, ask yourself this simple question: "What does she need to connect to, and what does she need help disconnecting from?" (Yapko, personal communication, 2005). This question—which is critical to answer when treating anxiety—is helpful with other issues, as you'll see when we discuss, for example, depression or medical treatment.

Hypnotic suggestions should introduce the idea of stepping back and getting a different look at one's own thoughts, symptoms, or resources. Teaching a child to dissociate in a helpful way from the habits of her anxious brain or body is essential. Again, we're not denying or suppressing the presence of these thoughts, feelings, or sensations, but creating a healthy separation. Children can be coached to step back from their anxious symptoms, to recognize and name them, and then actively decide what's worthy of their attention. Once some distance is created, the ability to see the thoughts or sensations as "background noise," "thought bugs that bug me," or "tricky intrusive thoughts" allow the child to develop a different response.

This skill is particularly helpful when dealing with OCD, where the content of the thoughts (a vast field of seemingly endless variety) is always irrelevant, but the process is the same. Even young children are able to see the OCD as a bossy part that will show up and say things that feel important, but are just noise or tricks. You may choose to teach a child, "Go to a special place in your imagination where you can feel powerful and talk back to your worry/bossy part/ OCD" as a way to experience positive dissociation.

Sabrina was a young girl who loved to go camping with her family. Consequently, she created her own "power tent." In her imagination she would practice climbing in, zipping down the flaps, and focusing on what she knew about her OCD's tricks. Then she could "come out of the tent and be ready for its bossy games." Kaiser (2014) described using and then imagining looking through binoculars backward as a way to create distance and shrink the size of overwhelming, global worries. John March's book for kids and parents, *Talking Back to OCD*, offers multiple CBT strategies for responding differently to the "hiccups" of OCD. Although March doesn't use the term *hypnosis*, his tools for chilling out or letting OCD "float by without focusing your attention on it" (2007, p. 159) can certainly be incorporated into a hypnotic intervention. As I said earlier, the use of breathing or calming strategies, when presented as a helpful bridge to connect to one's strengths and reboot, can be very useful. When young Sabrina went into her tent, she used several slowing-down tools to focus her attention and create the right climate inside for the job at hand (Yapko, 2014).

Several years ago I worked with Trina, a 20-year-old elite runner who was on the verge of making her nation's Olympic track team. As a child, she had vomited during the second half of her race. Now, many years later, she would back off as she passed the halfway mark, the very spot in the race where her coach wanted her to pick up the pace. She described the pattern easily: as she approached the second half of the course, the memory of that event would pop into her head, and she would slow down, remembering how embarrassing and awful it was. What was she too connected to? The memory of a single incident that happened 8 years before. What was she disconnected from? Both the present moment when she needed to pick up her pace and her bigger goal of making it to the Olympics.

Our hypnosis sessions involved suggestions that helped her remember and then activate her already developed ability to effectively connect or ignore. Anyone who has trained at that level knows how to dissociate from immediate discomfort and focus on the larger goal. How many miserable practices had she endured? How many times had she wanted to sleep in, but dragged herself out of bed at dawn instead? Per her report, she routinely filtered out distractions at meets (other events, other runners, loud noises, discomforts like rainy weather).

The posthypnotic suggestion reiterated this ability, while making the appearance of her vomiting memory predictable and boring:

You have so many memories of so many laps and races . . . and many of those memories you routinely forget . . . or just occasionally remember. . . . So when you next approach that home stretch, you can expect that memory to pop up in a routine way . . . just as you told me you expect your lungs to burn and your feet to push off the track. . . . This one thought is simply a blip between breaths . . . in the distance . . . so much farther away than the finish line you're driving toward.

Of note here: teaching Trina relaxation skills to deal with her anxiety wasn't going to work, as it showed up in the middle of an intensely physical race.

This skill can be particularly helpful when addressing phobias, either resulting from a specific event or not. The phobic reaction often becomes increasingly global in nature, despite the fact that the stimulus is specific. For example, a specific fear of vomiting can result in a widespread avoidance of anything that is connected to vomit, including school, certain foods, and anyone who may have vomited recently. A fear of bees may result in a child refusing to leave the house as soon as flowers start to bloom. Cognitively, the child amplifies the fear with catastrophic predictions of what will happen if he were to face the feared object or circumstance. Again, even though the content is specific, the process is predictable. Hypnosis can help develop the "content-free" ability to step back and discriminate between:

- Past events and current circumstances
- Perceived inadequacies and a demonstrated ability to problem solve or cope
- Realistic danger (or the need for caution) and a habitual global avoidance

Kevin, for example, developed a dog phobia after being severely bitten by a neighbor's dog when he was 9. Everyone understood Kevin's fear, and for two years had helped protect him from any encounters with dogs. Kevin himself told me he loved dogs, but now didn't trust "any dog. . . . I don't know what they will do." He and his parents sought help because he was avoiding activities that he loved. He wanted to be "his regular self again." Prior to being bitten, Kevin was around dogs frequently.

Our sessions focused not on relaxing around dogs, or letting go of his worries about dogs, but on reclaiming a skill he had practiced routinely and automatically before the dog bite: discriminating between dogs to approach, dogs to leave alone, and dogs to actively avoid. The initial induction and response set offered Kevin general ideas about how "we tell the difference," for example, how cave men learned to tell the difference between useless plants and healthy plants, and how when he skied he learned to determine when a slope was too easy, too hard, or appropriate for his skills. Working from general to specific, we moved toward the process of assessing safety versus danger, at first staying away from the content of dogs. Once this process was amplified, Kevin then imagined—by looking at the far wall in my office with his eyes open—how he would determine the different categories of dogs. His karate teacher, for example, had an old, friendly golden retriever that could barely get up to greet him with a wagging tail. Kevin had been refusing to go to his karate lessons because of his global assessment that "there is a dog there." Suggestions made throughout our time together supported his ability to tell the difference, and to slowly but surely use his ability to observe dogs to make his decisions. This leads us to our final frame with anxiety: action counts.

ACTION COUNTS

Because the hallmark of anxiety is avoidance, successful coping must ultimately include stepping into the feared situation. The previous sections have outlined skills that equip children to take this action—and action they must take. We want children to adopt this stance: "Anxiety and worry are normal, and I will feel uncertain and uncomfortable as I move forward into action." Hypnosis, as always, can be used as a way to rehearse how to use the skills, and to internalize the benefits of adopting this offensive (stepping toward) rather than defensive (backing away) approach.

When introducing the concept of action over avoidance, focus on building momentum in the direction of learning by doing. Your response set might describe the many things we can only learn by doing: swimming, riding a bike, reading. I often say to children,

> *I can sit here in my office and imagine flying a plane . . . oper-*
> *ating all the controls . . . taking off and landing . . . zooming*
> *through the clouds . . . but imagine how silly it would be . . . if*
> *I applied for a job at American Airlines . . . and told them I was*
> *a pilot . . . because I learned sitting here in this chair!*

This important frame builds on everything you've done so far to help the anxious child approach uncertainty in an engaged, proactive way. While anxiety globally announces, "You can't handle it," children develop self-confidence and a sense of mastery when they experiment, try, fail, and succeed. The message is this: "Of course you'll feel awkward and clumsy when you try something new! Of course you're going to make mistakes! You may even decide that something isn't for you, like roller coasters or scary movies or playing the oboe, but let action and experimenting guide your decisions. Give yourself a chance to move through the discomfort of not knowing. . . . Let yourself discover what comes next."

After our preparation together, Kevin needed to practice his dog-assessing skills in order to gain confidence. He also needed to experience the anxious response his body would have when he saw a dog. No amount of reassurance from adults or suggestions that he calm down was going to make him completely comfortable as he moved forward. Hypnosis with anxiety is a way to rehearse the use of skills out in the world, expecting the thoughts and feelings to arrive, and practicing a different response. Kevin did this as he looked at my wall, just as Benjamin talked to the waitress "in his mind" as he learned to manage his selective mutism in Chapter 4.

Kevin and I agreed that he would venture back into places where dogs might be: the soccer field, his karate teacher's studio, and his cousin's house. We role-played and hypnotically rehearsed how he would use his skills and then made a recording of statements that activated his discrimination strategies. Importantly, the goal was to assess the dogs and his body's reactions, without the need to reflexively avoid either:

> As you step forward and notice a dog, your smart and experienced brain will look at the dog's behavior. . . . Your smart brain might also notice how your heart is pumping, or how your hands feel shaky . . . all things that your body will do as you learn and relearn. . . . You can pay attention to slowing down if you like . . . slowing down your breathing for a moment . . . your thoughts . . . knowing the difference between then and now . . . and just observing for a bit . . . understanding the signals . . . giving yourself a few minutes to connect to what you know about dogs . . . all the different things you know . . . connecting to what you want in your life . . . even while you feel your body getting used to the idea . . . and reminding yourself . . . "Look at me! I'm doing it!"

Using hypnosis to support his new cognitive and behavioral skills, Kevin learned to reappraise and respond differently to both his body's reactions and his global thoughts about dogs. He asked himself, "What do I need to pay attention to, and what can just be in the background?" Then, by adopting an active stance, he learned to step into his ability to appraise dogs as a "kid who loves dogs, but was bitten by *one* dog." His past experience mattered and would be a part of his current appraisal, but not the only salient factor.

This chapter illustrates that your hypnotic interventions must be designed to bolster effective therapeutic strategies (Yapko, 2012; Golden, 2012). Although some studies seek to compare hypnosis with children with other therapeutic interventions like CBT (for example, Liossi & Hatira, 1999), I don't know how we can do hypnosis with a child, separate from doing therapy. Is not your hypnotic intervention the means by which you offer your therapy? We don't treat anxiety (or anything) by doing hypnosis. Instead, we figure out what a child—in this chapter, the anxious child—needs, and then embrace hypnosis as an effective and creative partner in the introduction, teaching, and experiencing of these skills.

As we move on to discuss depression, you will certainly see the overlaps in the frames we introduced with anxiety. Children's problems don't tend to fall into neat diagnostic categories, as the next chapters will illustrate.

CHAPTER 7

Hypnosis and Depression

Opportunities for Prevention
and Skill Building

*I*n the 25 years I have been a therapist, changes in the recognition
and treatment of depression in children and teens have been enor-
mous. Depression in children went from a status of nonexistent in
the 1950s and 1960s to being identified as the number one cause
of illness and disability in adolescents, defined as those ages 10–19
(World Health Organization, 2014). How we define and best treat
childhood depression remains up for debate. One need only look at
the numerous theories, studies, and models available to grasp the
complexity that surrounds it. Sadly, despite the increase in recognition, treatment options, medications, and information available to
health care providers and the public, we have yet to find a way to
loosen depression's grip on today's youth.

What are some of the many theories and treatment approaches?

As discussed in Chapter 4, cognitive behaviorists look at the relationship between events, thoughts, and reactions, targeting the automatic beliefs that support one's negative and hopeless conclusions (Seligman, 1989, 1995, 2011; Nolen-Hoeksema, Girgus, & Seligman, 1992; Weems et al., 2001, 2007; Beck, 1976; Beck et al., 1979). Kaslow and colleagues (1992) developed the Cognitive Triad Inventory for Children based on Beck's (1976) negative triad in adults, and found that both depressed and depressed-anxious children—like depressed adults—had a negative view of themselves, their world, and the future.

The question of how childhood depression relates to anxiety and other diagnoses has become a prominent issue, as anxiety frequently precedes depression in children, and the mechanisms of both are similar (Trosper, Buzzella, Bennett, & Ehrenreich, 2009; Dozois & Westra, 2004; Brown & Barlow, 2009; Kaslow et al., 1992; McLaughlin & Nolen-Hoeksema, 2011). Based on the predictable course of childhood anxiety into adolescent depression, some suggest a model of treatment that moves away from diagnostic categories, and toward a more general and earlier skill-building approach. For example, Angus Thompson (2012) questioned how we are defining and distinguishing childhood anxiety and depression in his article "Childhood Depression Revisited: Indicators, Normative Tests, and Clinical Course":

- How do we understand the oft-described differences between the presentations of childhood, adolescent, and adult depression?
- How do we distinguish between anxiety and depression in children, when the two appear to be so intertwined?
- In looking at the effectiveness of the Childhood Depression Inventory (Kovacs, 1992) in measuring depression, Thompson wrote that it "measures something very well that appears to be important" but does not discriminate well between depression and other diagnoses, particularly anxiety.

Equally important in understanding childhood depression are family and social connections (Wagner & Ambrosini, 2001;

McArdle, 2007; Nolen-Hoeksema et al., 1995). A 5-year meta-analysis on the link between maternal depression and childhood depression supported the researchers' contention that maternal depression is the most consistent and well-replicated risk factor for major depressive disorders in children (Mendes et al., 2012). Parental conflict, overinvolvement, and restriction of autonomy predicted depression in teens (Yap, Pilkington, Ryan, & Jorm, 2014). Miriam Tisher (2007), a family therapist and developer of the Children's Depression Scale, described the numerous and evolving conceptions of childhood depression—from biological to developmental to sociological—and the impact that different conceptualizations have on one's treatment approach. She emphasized the importance of recognizing a family's blocked communication, and the need for emotional expressiveness to help hear and heal the hurt.

Depressed adolescents use social withdrawal as a coping strategy, adding to their sadness, isolation, and risk of suicide (Campbell-Sills & Barlow, 2007; Ivarsson, Gillberg, Arvidsson, & Broberg, 2002). On the flip side, a program that focuses on parental interaction with depressed preschool children has been successful in reducing depressive symptoms (Luby, Lenze, & Tillman, 2012). Teens who have strong supports at school with teachers and peers have less depression (Joyce & Early, 2014) and one study found that teens' successful self-help interventions to deal with their depression included social support and behavioral activation (Wisdom & Barker, 2006).

With depression, prevention is again a key component to limit suffering. Research shows that subthreshold depressive symptoms often precede a major depressive episode (Brent, Birmaher, Kolko, Baugher, & Bridge, 2001) and that the risk of a future depressive episode increases with each sequential bout (Teasedale et al., 2000; Nolen-Hoeksema et al., 1992). These subthreshold symptoms often go untreated, but if addressed could be essential in interrupting depression's chronic course (Dozois & Westra, 2004). Importantly, hypnosis is conducive to the positive skill building inherent in a prevention framework.

Finally, the neuroscience of depression, and more broadly the relationship between temperament, genes, life events, and pediatric mental illness, create interesting possibilities as we learn more about epigenetics, brain plasticity, and gene expression. Although most of us are familiar (and comfortable) with the concept that certain genetic temperaments or predispositions put people at risk for certain disorders—for example, behaviorally inhibited children have greater risks for both anxiety and depression (Biederman et al., 1990; Caspi, Moffitt, Newman, & Silva, 1996)—the field of translational developmental neuroscience looks at the likely bidirectional relationship between genes and environment, with both positive and negative outcomes. The National Advisory Mental Health Council defined this new field thus: "This new collaborative science will explore and explain how the healthy brain develops, how neurodevelopmental processes go awry in mental illness, and how to re-position these neurodevelopmental processes on a healthy trajectory" (2008, p. 6).

It's easy to feel overwhelmed and confused by the many theories and as yet unanswered questions about children and depression. Our understanding of depression in children is evolving and changing, particularly the correlations between anxiety and depression. The question to address in this book on pediatric hypnosis is this: how can we effectively use hypnosis to improve the present and future of a depressed child, and thus prevent a chronic struggle that continues from childhood to adolescence to adulthood?

There are no controlled research studies on the use of hypnosis for depressed children. Several texts and chapters (Kohen, 2013; Yapko, 2012; Kohen & Olness, 2011; Kohen & Murray, 2006) recognize the value of hypnosis as a way to interrupt a child's negative trance, offer hope, teach self-soothing, and build ego strength. Yapko wrote of the benefit of using hypnosis to teach preventative skills to a depressed child, including emotional management, relaxation, and critical thinking: "The more complex uses of hypnosis to teach specific skills (e.g. problem solving, decision making) holds even greater potential for meaningful intervention with at-risk kids" (2012, p. 490).

Painting with the broadest of strokes, our goal is to build (or rebuild) the skills that help children create positive relationships, solve problems flexibly, and chose action over rumination. And we must often do this in a context of loss, conflict, illness, and rejection. No easy task, but this is where the positive psychology of hypnosis steps in—the ability to shift a frame and offer something different, and to perhaps alter the trajectory of development by altering genetic expression (Rossi & Rossi, 2008). The severity of life events matters, of course, but as Jerome Kagan observes, "the private interpretations of stressful events and the accompanying feelings are more significant causes of symptoms than the events the camera records" (2013, p. 230).

Let's again take the broad frames from Chapter 4, combine them with what we know about successful treatment strategies, and create interventions that work for the child in front of you. You'll discover, as I did in the writing of this chapter, that the frames are more overlapping than distinct, both among themselves and with the interventions used to help with anxiety.

EXPERIENCE IS VARIABLE: QUICKER TO HOPE

Aristotle is quoted as saying, "Youth is easily deceived because it is quick to hope." If you've been in the presence of a depressed child, you only wish that were the case. When a child concludes that his current circumstances cannot and will not change, he has likely lost track of his motivation, flexibility, and, quite often, his trust that adults can do anything to help. This stable attributional style—a rigid perception that life will stay this awful—is a defining pattern of depression (Yapko, 1992, 2010b). And because apathy is such a sad and dangerous place for a child's mind to be stuck, you must cultivate hope and positive expectancy from the start (M.D. Yapko, 2006, 2010b, 2010c; Lynn & Kirsch, 2006). After all, a hopeless child needs a reason to engage in the process of his own healing, a reason to shift from apathy to, at the very least, thinking, "Well, maybe something can be different. Maybe there is something that will help."

How do we do this? Just as with anxious children, the key is to emphasize malleability, particularly about the present and the future. We want to introduce the idea that even though many external and past events are not in our control and cannot be altered, some important elements of our experience are changeable—and we should have some say in that.

Planting the seed of an idea within a child and his parents that this experience might not be permanent as time moves forward is critical. Not surprisingly, a 2013 study found that when people with significant depression were told that their depression was biochemical and genetic, they were more pessimistic about their prognosis for recovery. But when people were given psychoeducation about the malleability of gene effects and neurochemistry, their hopefulness and optimism increased (Lebowitz, Ahn, & Nolen-Hoeksema, 2013). Furthermore, a pessimistic explanatory style was shown to be a significant predictor of depression as a child aged, more so than negative life events (Nolen-Hoeksema et al., 1992). How many children and their parents have been told that "depression is like diabetes," that it is genetic and permanent, or that they should plan to be on medication for the rest of their lives? How does this impact one's view of the future, and motivation to change it? Such permanent, pessimism-bolstering suggestions are powerful—and currently reinforced by multiple sources.

There is a distinction to be made between an anxious child's and a depressed child's relationship to certainty and the future. For anxious children, certainty is the elusive goal. They strive to eliminate uncertainty and need to be taught how to handle its inevitable arrival. ("I don't know what's going to happen and I can't handle that! Tell me what will happen!") In contrast, a depressed child will often focus on the bleak certainty of his future. ("I know what will happen at school tomorrow . . . more of the same. . . . I can predict with certainty how awful I will feel.") Where do they intersect? Both see the future as dark, based on either its overwhelming unpredictability or its overwhelming bleakness.

Hope for a depressed child begins with your message that change is inevitable, and is strengthened by his (tentative) willingness to consider that the future has something to offer. From that tentative platform, you can address the patterns that support depression, such as perfectionism, permanence, and rumination (Nolen-Hoeksema et al., 1992; Davis & Nolen-Hoeksema, 2000; Roelofs et al., 2009; McLaughlin & Nolen-Hoeksema, 2011; Michl, McLaughlin, Shepherd, & Nolen-Hoeksema, 2013) and of course offer alternatives.

For younger children, teaching emotional regulation and expression can be coupled with the message that feelings change. As mentioned above, young children are likely to express their emotional pain as anxiety, anger, irritability, and somatic complaints, not just sadness. Children have difficulty articulating their emotional states, and thus the simple and concrete intervention of helping a child express her emotional state and then shift from one state to another is useful. Because younger children tend to be more somatic in their expression of symptoms, teaching a child how to alter her physical body (e.g., from tight to loose, from busy to quiet, from light to heavy) demonstrates on multiple levels the ability to change.

Induction

As Kohen and Murray (2006) pointed out, depressed children are often already focused hypnotically on their negative feelings and the narrative that nothing will change. Acknowledging this focus and introducing the possibility of change is done by simply stating, "I know you've been thinking a lot about [problem], so much so that it probably feels like you can't think of anything else sometimes. Kids tell me that it's nice to take a break from that. Even just taking a few minutes to pay attention to something different. . . ."

From here, any age-appropriate suggestion that creates an actual shift in attention—while hinting at the more general ability to separate from one's immediate experience—will do, utilizing both what you know about the child and what's happening in the environment.

Sometimes I can get lost in all the colors and designs of my rug. . . . What do you see? It's funny how everyone finds different things in there. . . .

Would you like to draw together? [The content of the drawing then begins the conversation. . . .]

I wonder if you can notice all the sounds happening outside the office. . . . You can close your eyes and just listen for a bit. . . . Sometimes it's surprising how much is going on out there. . . .

Do you have any places you like to go in your imagination? Any thoughts that take you away on a little mental vacation?

I know you've been working hard lately, feeling and thinking about so many important things. . . . I hear how stuck you feel in those thoughts and feelings . . . and how nice it would be to move forward into a different way of thinking. . . . If you'd like, you can sit back and just let your thinking slow down, or simply focus on the sound of my voice, a different voice. . . .

Building a Response Set: Hope, Change, Shifts

The response set then suggests in gentle ways that change is inevitable, and that although the past has already happened, we don't need to be stuck in its mud. The goal is to portray the future as malleable and the present state (emotional or otherwise) as temporary or changeable (Yapko, 2001, 2010a, 2010b). We are going after the rigidity and hopelessness that fuels apathy and planting seeds for future action and mastery. This is particularly important for children who may have no access to memories of feeling good and little historical context to suggest that anything could be different. Examples of positive experiences might be discussed with parents ahead of time, then delicately seeded into the session. Depressed kids have much to gain from exposure to an optimistic, future-oriented outlook. The comedian George Burns once said, "I look to the future because that's where I'm going to spend the rest of my life."

For younger children, a simple, engaging experience of feeling different (and your empathy as you help get them there) can be powerful. The entire hypnosis session may consist of a few sentences that introduce the idea of change, coupled with an experience or story that illustrates this very thing (Kuttner, 1988). Charlotte Reznick (2009) suggests having a child draw an outline of her body, close her eyes, and imagine where feelings are in her body, and then draw them on her body picture. The use of different colors, shapes, and characters all help make the feelings visible and ultimately changeable (as you'll see with the story of Derrick, below).

Here are some additional examples of response sets that move the child toward the ideas of malleability and change, as it relates to the future emotional states or perceptions (remember, the examples progress from younger to older):

Have you ever gone into a shoe store and seen the tiny shoes for the babies and toddlers? Can you imagine that your feet once fit into shoes that small? And then you walk over to the men's department and see the giant sneakers and work boots . . . and you can't imagine your feet being that big some day. . . .

I wonder how many feelings a kid could have in a day. And how many different reasons he might have to have those feelings. . . . Mad at his brother for eating the last waffle . . . then happy to see some friends on the bus . . . then worried about the quiz in math . . . and proud when he knew some answers . . . sad when a friend was mean . . . then tired when his head finally hit the pillow . . . so many in a day. . . . [With a younger child you could draw the faces or expressions, or have a feelings chart as a visual guide. Remember, young children often have difficulties articulating or naming their emotions with words; instead, they may mention pains or physical symptoms.]

Imagine if George Washington or Benjamin Franklin showed up today . . . all the things they'd see. . . . They would recognize the sun and the moon and the stars in the sky . . . but television? . . . Smartphones? . . . Frozen yogurt machines? . . . Washington and Franklin couldn't imagine what the world would look like today . . . and they might be delighted or surprised . . . even shocked! . . . But they were inventors who understood change . . . then and now. . . . People today and back in colonial times . . . are always coming up with new ideas and inventions . . . some that work and some that don't . . . but their eyes and ears and brains . . . stay open . . . on the lookout for what might be next. . . .

Interventions and Suggestions

Your interventions continue to build on this theme of malleability, shaking loose the child's internal focus on feelings of helplessness and hopelessness. Rubin Battino's 2007 article about brief therapy said it well: "Clients come to you because they are stuck: they either have one response to a given stimulus, or one interpretation of that stimulus. Your job is to provide them with choices (plural!) with respect to response and interpretation" (p. 21). Below I offer several examples of how rigidity leaves its mark, and how to offer, as Battino suggests, alternative interpretations.

The question to keep in the forefront of your thinking: How do I help this child believe that his current state is temporary and that his thoughts, perceptions, emotions, and reactions can change? How do I help him find hope?

Changing Feelings

As I have said, the elements of hypnotic interventions with kids are often free-flowing, especially with younger children where no formal process occurs. Derrick, for example, was 5 when his mother was diagnosed with cancer. He worried (understandably) throughout her treatment, but now she was months past treatment and cancer free. He was still, he told me, "sad when I am away from her. She is happy she is better, but I'm staying sad."

My goal was to help Derrick move into this different phase of his life where mom's cancer was gone and her recovery was solid, a phase where there was every reason to be optimistic.

You are 6, and already you know that life is full of changes, don't you? People change! Their hair changes and their eye-sight changes and their jobs change. Sometimes they go from well to sick to well again, just like Mom. And let's think about how you've changed! You used to be 5 and now you're 6. You are so much bigger and smarter than when we met. . . . You know so many new things! But did you know that sometimes even when things change and people change, even when moms get better, feelings can get stuck? It happens, to kids and to grownups. Maybe we can draw a picture that might help us see changing feelings instead of stuck feelings.

Derrick loved to draw. As he intently went to work, we narrated his story together.

D: This is Derrick when Mom had cancer. He was sad and
     worried.
L: Of course he was. It was a sad and worried time.
D: This is Derrick when Mom was better.
L: Did Sad stick around?
D: Yes, he did.
L: Is there something Derrick can say to Sad?
D: Then Derrick told Sad that it was okay to go. Here's me with a
     sword and some armor, showing Sad I'm strong.
L: It's okay if Sad comes back for a visit, don't you think?
D: Maybe, but then Happy will have to get bigger.
L: You just want Sad to stay smaller for now?
D: Yes, I don't need a big Sad right now.
L: I like that plan. That makes sense.

Derrick's parents reported that multiple mornings over the next few weeks, Derrick jumped onto his parents' bed and asked his dad to "be the Sad" and have a sword fight with him. Dad played his role well, falling to Derrick's dramatic attacks, announcing that he would be quiet for now, but he might show up again some day. Apparently, there was a lot of laughter all around.

Hope as the First (of Many) Steps

Older children, particularly teens, often arrive for psychotherapy with several issues to address or a history of past treatment. They may have been in therapy before, carry the baggage of multiple diagnoses, or have been struggling on their own while resisting any help. Family, peer, academic, and emotional struggles often come tangled together. In order to engage such tired-out teens in treatment, they must conclude that you have something different to offer, or, if new to treatment, find hope that this new and unfamiliar thing (be it therapy in general or hypnosis with you in particular) is actually worth the effort. An intervention that creates hope—necessary to get them coming back—is a frontline focus in what will likely be a multistep process. If they have come to you specifically looking to do hypnosis, then some expectancy and interest may already be present. (Use this card well.)

The induction, be it formal or informal, can be a simple invitation to "have an experience that will start the process of feeling better and get you where you want to be" and may involve any of the techniques that introduce a shift in attention toward a different experience.

The response set, like the examples above, paves the way for your suggestions with truisms about the experiences of trying something for the first time and those moments of discovery:

Have you ever really watched a person or an animal react to something new? . . . How the body and the brain respond to a novel experience? . . . Kids reading Harry Potter for the first time. . . . YouTube is filled with videos of puppies going down a staircase for the first time . . . and babies hearing silly noises and giggling with surprise . . . or people recovering their hearing and crying with joy. . . .

The session continues with a focus on how noticing and using one's own strengths and resources—combined with flexibility, curiosity, and the ability to learn new things—leads to changes in the present and the future. Age progression techniques that help a child imagine a different future and reactivate the process of discovery are essential and should be woven throughout (Yapko, 2010b, 2010c, 2012; Lynn & Kirsch, 2006).

So, here you are, in the midst of a new experience . . . and as you listen to the sound of my voice . . . you might be thinking about how many voices you've heard over the years. . . . A person can get a variety of opinions about the same problem . . . or the same old solutions to a variety of problems . . . but it's that interesting idea or perspective that catches your ear . . . sparks your thinking . . . how we can see things in a new way . . . or interpret an old problem from a different angle. . . . The chef that combines ingredients like no one else has done before . . . the designer who can transform a room by removing a wall . . . and sometimes the shifts aren't always dramatic . . . or even visible to others . . . a change in the pace of your breath . . . or where you put your focus. . . .

Some people do the same things over and over . . . and some people just don't know of any other options . . . but I wonder . . . as you sit here . . . what experience you have with doing things differently . . . or thinking about things in a new way . . . or what you have learned. . . . Big things and small things . . . like how to say the alphabet . . . and how to read . . . or how to use a new phone or app. . . . How automatic that seems to you now . . . and combined with some confident feelings about what you already know . . . because I know that you know quite a lot . . . you might have some ideas about what you still want

*to learn. . . . You can't know everything yet. . . . There's so
much out there. . . .*

Simply check in by saying,

*I've been talking for awhile, and you've been listening. I wonder
if you have anything you'd like to share. Any words or thoughts
that caught your attention? You can stay focused and relaxed
as you speak. . . .*

After this interaction (adjusting and using the feedback given),
offer the posthypnotic suggestion, focusing on how things can be
different:

*As you move through your daily life . . . going to school, hang-
ing out with friends, even dealing with frustration . . . I wonder
how often you'll notice something new in your environment or
your interactions . . . when you're home or at school, how you
might see things through a different set of eyes . . . maybe in
the eye of the hurricane . . . or say things with a different set of
words . . . even if it's just what you say to yourself . . . and who
knows what might happen from there. . . . I heard you when
you said that you've been feeling lousy for a long time. . . .
Maybe as the next few weeks unfold . . . you'll notice moments
here and there of less lousy . . . maybe because you do something new or hear something curious or funny . . . and I'll look
forward to hearing about what you notice . . . what gets your
attention on the inside and the outside. . . .*

Time of Wonder, an illustrated book written in 1957 by well-
known children's author Robert McCloskey, tells the story of a children's summer on an island in Maine. A passage in this book is a

185

wonderful example of a change in perspective and could be incorporated into a session with a depressed child or teen:

> *A book called* Time of Wonder . . . *talks about all the changes*
> *that happened over a summer on an island in Maine . . . and*
> *the book talks to the children on the island . . . and what they*
> *discovered the night after a hurricane. . . . I'd like to read you*
> *a page from the book. . . . [Or with a younger child, read the*
> *book together.]*
>
> > The next morning you awaken to an unaccustomed light
> > made by a frosty coating of salt on all the windows. And
> > out-of-doors in the gentle morning lie reminders of yester-
> > day's hurricane. Fallen and broken trees are everywhere—
> > on the terrace, on the path—blocking your way at every
> > turn. You cannot walk on familiar paths and trails, but you
> > can explore the tops of giant fallen trees, and walk on trunks
> > and limbs where no one ever walked before. (McCloskey,
> > 1957, p. 34)

Importantly, parents should continue to carry this torch of perspective change by reading such a story with a young child at home. The ritual reinforces and integrates this new way of looking at experiences for the child—and perhaps spills over to the parent, who may also benefit from the same shift in perspective.

Perfectionism

Not surprisingly, perfectionism has been correlated with increased levels of depression and distress in children (Hewitt et al., 2002), more acute depression and higher rates of suicidality in teens ages 12–17 (Jacobs et al., 2009), and higher levels of anxiety in children (e.g., Flett, Coulter, Hewitt, & Nepon, 2011; Mitchell et al., 2013). As discussed in Chapter 6, the inability to handle change, uncertainty, and mistakes are all rigid patterns that impede growth. Perfectionism, a pinnacle of internal rigidity, is a setup for feeling badly about oneself. The self-talk of a perfectionist is unforgiving and critical. The good news is that brief treatment has been effective in changing perfectionism in teens, with some indications that perfectionism is more malleable in younger populations than with adults (Jacobs et al., 2009).

Perfectionism is a two-timer with anxiety and depression. It demands that the future go exactly as planned ("I can't handle things not working out the way I imagine!"), but destroys hope by setting the bar impossibly high ("I'll never be perfect . . . all this work for nothing. . . . Why do I even bother?"). Think about how to create interventions that show children both the inevitability and value of imperfection. How are mistakes a part of learning, sports, great inventions? How do things improve by trying, failing, and then trying again? Pencils have erasers; computers have delete keys; and people have apologies. Athletes strike out, drop passes, foul out, and miss shots on goal. Actors, dancers, and musicians rehearse and rehearse, and still sing a wrong note or miss a step. Then they make adjustments, using the input from a recent performance to make improvements.

Here are some ideas. The induction can offer many choices and the opportunity to "try different ways of sitting, and you can listen with your eyes open or with them closed. . . . Adjust along the way if something doesn't work." (You as the therapist can change your mind about where you're going to sit, for example, or purposely make a mistake of some sort.)

The response set builds momentum with truisms about how the definition of perfect keeps changing.

The more we experiment and fail and succeed, the more we discover and the more options we have. . . . We used to think the perfect way to travel was by foot, then by horse and carriage, then by car, and then by jet. . . . And now we have so

*many options. . . . Some still like to go by horse while others
are waiting to take a rocket to Mars! . . . So many different
paths . . . and many ways to get there. . . .*

You can then continue to play around with the idea of "perfect,"
suggesting the child think about the many definitions of the perfect
dessert, the perfect vacation, the perfect birthday party; the perfect
song or the perfect bedtime; the perfect car, the perfect dress, the
perfect TV show.

*And one person might think the perfect dessert is chocolate
cake, while another wants apple pie, and the perfect vacation
for you might be a trip to a water park or a beach, while your
friend imagines skiing in the mountains. . . . And when you
were 4 the perfect toys were blocks and crayons and trucks,
but that has changed over the years, hasn't it? . . . And even if
there is a perfect answer, like knowing that 8 plus 7 is 15 . . .
there are many ways to get there . . . using your fingers and
your toes, or a calculator, or pieces of bubble gum, or asking
your brother . . . and probably making some mistakes along the
way . . . which is perfectly understandable. . . .*

Then get more specific, helping the child to see how he has changed
and learned while making mistakes and adjustments in the process, checking in and asking about his own experiences of learning,
changing, messing up. Older children may know of historical figures
that discovered things through errors or experimentation. Such stories and metaphors are everywhere.

The posthypnotic suggestion then connects the concept of inevitable (and even positive) imperfection to the child's own world:

*And so I wonder how you'll smile when you notice what's
imperfect about that goofy dog you love . . . and how many*

*silly mistakes your friends make . . . and you end up laughing
. . . or how your teacher corrects you when working on a project. . . . What would it be like to watch some blooper videos
on YouTube? . . . And how will you slowly begin to change your
own view of perfect, and notice too how you can talk to yourself
in a different way, giving yourself some room to grow . . . along
with some room for mistakes?*

Rumination and Perseveration: How to Stay Stuck

Rumination is the process, through thoughts and behaviors, of consistently focusing on how badly one feels and then analyzing why
one feels so badly. Research done primarily by Susan Nolen-Hoeksema and her colleagues shows that ruminators are at greater risk for
depression, and have longer and more intense episodes of depression, but have great difficulty problem solving or taking action that
would improve their circumstances or change their mood (Nolen-
Hoeksema, 1991; Butler & Nolen-Hoeksema, 1994; Lyubomirsky
& Nolen-Hoeksema, 1993; Lyubomirsky, Caldwell, & Nolen-Hoeksema, 1998). A study by Davis and Nolen-Hoeksema looked at
rumination as a "manifestation of a more general tendency toward
cognitive inflexibility, or perseveration" (2000, p. 701). They confirmed in ruminators a level of cognitive inflexibility that made it
difficult to shift attention or adjust coping strategies—even when
negative feedback from the environment told them, "What you're
doing is not working!"

Several researchers have looked at how ruminating in children
and teens predicts depression and anxiety. Hilt, Armstrong, and
Essex (2012) examined early childhood risk factors that create ruminating teens. Adolescent ruminators, they found, were correlated
with (1) overcontrolling parents, perhaps resulting in the suppression of affect; (2) the overexpression of feelings like sadness, guilt,
and embarrassment by parents; (3) a high negative affect in the child;

and (4) low levels of effortful control, measured by the inability to follow directions and maintain focus on a neutral stimulus. Hilt and Pollak (2013) reported that children as young as 9 show patterns of ruminating that lead to negative self-referential thoughts. While everyone does this at times, it was the inability to disengage from these thoughts that predicted problems for children.

Hypnosis offers us many options if our goal is to interrupt this thought pattern and refocus attention. It's important to note, however, that distraction is a helpful strategy when used in concert with other coping strategies such as problem solving, but not as a way to avoid or suppress discomfort (Trosper et al., 2009). Many have shared their ideas about how to disengage from ruminating thoughts by shifting or engaging, rather than suppressing. Lynn, Barnes, Deming, and Accardi, for example, described using hypnosis with ruminators as a way to "enhance mental agility" (2010, p. 205). Wells (2008) described attention-training techniques that switch attention away from ruminative thoughts to an awareness of sounds in the present environment. Roelofs et al. (2009) described several ways to help vulnerable children manage rumination with a goal of moving away from self-focused attention. These include active distraction, cognitive awareness and replacement of ruminative thoughts, and mindfulness or acceptance strategies that allow children to recognize and allow the thoughts, but not listen to or judge them.

To address rumination, create an absorbing, hypnotic experience—or several—that demonstrate how to:

- Externalize "the Ruminator" as a part of them that gets stuck, or repeats the same thing over and over, but doesn't help to solve the problem. Have fun creating a character that the child can see and hear.
- Notice and recognize when the Ruminator shows up and do a visual (or experiential) muting, shrinking, or changing the Ruminator in some way.

- Accept and hear the Ruminator; allow it to be there, but dismiss its message as unimportant or old news (as we did with anxiety). "There's my worry/ruminator part showing up again!"
- Shift focus to other activities or stimuli, for example, music, sounds outside (like birds, traffic, music) in order to cognitively interrupt the perseveration.
- Move into problem-solving mode, using mental rehearsal first with an active homework assignment to follow. Some kids like to create a "Problem Solver Partner" that shows up to help figure out what to do next.

ACTION COUNTS

Now that we have created hope, planted seeds that the future can be different, and addressed the paralyzing cognitive rigidity of perfectionism and rumination, we need to help the depressed child take some action. As discussed above, thinking has its limits. Ruminators think they're being productive, but in actuality they are spinning their wheels in cognitive mud. Susan Nolen-Hoeksema said it just right: "Our research clearly suggests that dysphoric people can get temporary relief from their mood, and more important, can go on to think more constructively and problem solve more effectively if they use positive distractors to get their minds off their ruminations for a while" (1998, p. 218). Positive distractors may include positive thoughts, but also include "getting people to get out of the house and do something active and constructive" (p. 218).

As you may remember from Chapter 4, the behavioral activation model emphasizes the need to engage in healthy behaviors rather than depressed behaviors in order to change negative patterns of thought and the resultant depressed feelings. Thus, in this model, action would precede cognitive shifts. In their treatment manual using behavioral activation for depression in adults, Lejuez and colleagues stated: "We suggest that negative thoughts and feelings often will change only after positive events and consequences are experienced more frequently. Said more simply, it is difficult to feel depressed and have low self-esteem if you are regularly engaging in activities that bring you a sense of pleasure and/or accomplishment" (2001, p. 261).

Acknowledging that more research needs to be done on the use of this specific model with younger adolescents and children (Ruggiero, Morris, Hopko, & Lejuez, 2007), the benefit of moving a distressed child into action, particularly toward greater social connection, is well supported (David-Ferndon & Kaslow, 2008) and an important part of cognitive-behavioral treatment. Depressed children have trouble doing, but they need positive, pleasurable experiences to contradict their negative and often avoidant patterns. Hypnotic interventions are themselves experiential, and can be used to rehearse and imagine future action like fun experiences, problem solving, and social interactions (Lynn & Kirsch, 2006; Lynn, Barnes, et al., 2010; Yapko, 2010b, 2010c). Sequentially, consider the option of putting the pleasurable experience first. Why not take a trip to the ice cream shop, the mall, or the pet store, and then follow up the concrete favorable experience with a hypnosis session that builds on the evidence that doing things can change your mood?

A focus on creating immediate positive experiences is particularly important for younger children who lack cognitive skills and whose depression is most strongly correlated to negative life events (Nolen-Hoeksema et al., 1992). The first place to start? Your interactions. Drawing pictures, role-playing, and making recordings all give you the opportunity to join powerful suggestions with an experience of fun. Engaging a parent in this—especially a depressed one—is great modeling, as well. (I talk more in depth about the role of parents in Chapter 10.)

*Let's make a list of five [or three or two] things you love to do
. . . or things you really want to do sometime. . . . Let's write
them down together . . . and then let's pick one and pretend
we're doing it. . . . Do you remember the last time you had fun?
Let's have fun thinking about and pretending we're having fun!*

You can substitute any positive experience: "Let's make a list of five
things . . ."

- That make you feel strong
- That you can do really well
- That made you feel proud of yourself

This can be adapted for use with older children as well. Invite
the child to join you in . . .

*Making some positive pathways . . . pathways in your brain that
need a little attention . . . positive imagination pathways that
can lead to doing pathways . . . a step at a time. . . .*

*It's important to keep those pathways open . . . because some-
times, when we're dealing with tough times and feelings, we
lose track of the things we most enjoy. . . . It's like we forget to
remember what makes us happy . . . and taking some time to
refresh those memories . . . to remind you of the brighter parts
of your life . . . and how to bring them back into your day . . .
can be a good experience. . . . Maybe it's something you used
to do a lot . . . or something you'd like to do soon . . . or something you've always wanted to try or see . . . and the depressed
[sad] part or pessimistic [grumpy] part of you might be chiming
in . . . telling you it won't happen . . . or you can't do that anymore . . . or whatever thought it throws your way . . . and that's
okay, too. . . . Those thoughts will show up . . . but even sitting*

*here and imagining what you like to do and want to do can help
open up those positive pathways. . . . Can you find something?
That's great. . . . Now let yourself get absorbed in it. . . . You
can tell me about it if you'd like . . . as you're seeing and hearing the details . . . or [for younger children] we can draw it. . . .*

Make sure you know what the child in front of you does well or
enjoys (from parents or teachers as needed), so that if he can't
retrieve anything, you can prompt him:

*I remember you telling me [or hearing] about you and fishing
. . . and how you like to go to that pond near your house. . . .
Maybe we can imagine going together . . . right now. . . . I'll
help get you started and then we can fill in the details. . . .*

After conversing about the experience, the posthypnotic suggestion with all ages then predicts taking action outside of the hypnotic,
imaginative rehearsal:

*Now that we've started clearing out the positive pathway in your
brain. . . . You might discover that the doing something fun or positive actually feels and sounds like a good idea . . . that your body
and your mind and your imagination are able to team up . . . and
take a few more steps in that direction . . . and it doesn't mean that
everything will be fine . . . or that you still don't have to deal with
those tough feelings at times, too . . . but taking a break . . . just
like we did today . . . to have some time to focus on some fun . . .
that's an idea worth chewing on . . . and it might feel different than
it did in the past . . . and that's okay. . . . Maybe the more you do
those fun things . . . the more it will feel like it used to . . . and like
many things as you are growing older, some things you will start to
like less, and some things you will start to like more . . . just like*

your Legos in the attic, and now your latest computer game. . . .

The follow-up to this session is an assignment to engage in some positive activity and then report back. Or, at the very least, the child starts by listening to the recording of the session, independently imagining an activity, or making concrete plans to engage in a pleasurable activity (Lynn, Barnes et al., 2010).

Dr. Martin Seligman, a driving force behind the positive psychology movement, has a simple exercise he calls What Went Well. Each evening children are asked to list three things that went well that day, and then to answer the question, "Why did this good thing happen to you?" In his 2011 book *Flourish*, Seligman describes the use of this exercise and others as part of the Penn Resiliency Program, designed to bring positive psychology and a strength-based approach into schools. (One kindergarten class started each morning with the exercise.) When Seligman gathered data both formally and informally from depressed adults who participated in the exercise daily, he found the impact on their depressive symptoms was significant and long lasting. This exercise creates an experience that encompasses all three broad frames: (1) good things do happen (experience is variable); (2) when you notice, write down, and report on positive things, you feel better, and you can connect the impact of actions on better outcomes (action counts); and (3) you can focus on the positive parts of your day-to-day life (the value of parts). An added bonus: the social reinforcement of hearing peers report on positive events. That's good modeling.

A Problem-Solving, Action-Taking Book

Alvah and Arvilla, by New Hampshire author Mary Lyn Ray, tells the story of two farmers who have been married for 31 years but have never taken a vacation because of the daily demands of running their farm. Arvilla dreams of seeing the Pacific Ocean, so she comes up with a plan to pack up all their belongings and animals and make the journey to California. After some convincing, she and Alvah plan and prepare and build a traveling farm of sorts that takes them across the country. They and their assortment of animal companions spend several days relaxing on the beach, and when they return home, spread the sand they collected to make their own tiny beach. The story illustrates persistence, creativity, partnership, and adventure. Arvilla may have been dreaming of a vacation for 31 years, but now she's going to make it happen. (Hopefully the child can choose to do what he likes before 31 years pass.)

THE VALUE OF PARTS: FLEXIBLY CONNECTING AND DISCONNECTING

As I'm sure you've noticed, many of the interventions already described in this chapter involve elements of parts. Helping to differentiate aspects of experiences, relationships, and oneself is necessary and inevitable when working with depressed children because they are so absorbed in their globally negative frame. They will recall negative information more readily when discussing past memories (Bishop, Dalgleish, & Yule, 2004) and predict ongoing negative outcomes as they look to the future. In fact, Reid, Salmon, and Lovibond (2006) found a general bias across all emotional disorders for attention to the negative.

And, as I said above, the section on parts in Chapter 6 is highly relevant to depressed children because of the overlap in cognitive patterns; so certainly review that section for ideas to use with depressed kids, as well.

I now describe a few additional ideas for incorporating the concept of parts using the frame of connection and disconnection. The issue of when to connect and when to disconnect is particularly relevant to depressed children because of their tendency to disconnect through isolation and withdrawal and internally overconnect to self-referential thoughts, feelings, and somatic symptoms. I then talk specifically about using compartments with grieving children.

Connecting to the Positive

Use hypnosis is to find the positive (a memory, a person, a strength, a place) and bring that resource into the child's current awareness. Kohen and Murray (2006) describe the affect bridge technique, an age regression strategy that prompts the child to go back to a time before she felt depressed, enjoy the memory, and then bring those positive feelings back to the present. Reid Wilson and I (2013) use the phrase "reminder bridges" to help children connect the resources used successfully in past to help with current challenges.

Distance From the Negative Part

Explain the pattern of negative bias in kid-friendly terms, for example, "Your brain is stuck in a habit of going back and remembering the lousy stuff, and sometimes doesn't even let you pay attention to the good stuff that is happening now!" Help the child create a part that represents his pattern of negative bias. One child decided to personify this habit into a part he called his Ya But part. We made a short recording together that prompted him to "go inside and travel through his day" until he found some positive experiences. We imagined Ya But showing up to complain about the negative and negate the positive. We didn't deny that some days were lousy, but decided that Ya But needed to be small and quiet so he could learn to pay attention to the good stuff and not only focus on the lousy stuff. Kay Thompson described her version of this as the "Yes, but . . ." device, and in more sophisticated language said the same thing: "This simple technique of redefinition allows the client to acknowledge the surface facts of a particular experience, but also recognize how to alter those facts with new information" (Kane & Olness, 2004, p. 63).

Connect to Others With Action

Depressed children (and anxious ones, too) don't feel like participating in activities and they use these feelings to guide their choices. This often leads to a cycle of isolation, low energy, and increased rumination. Hypnosis can help a child look at the role of feelings from what Yapko terms "a more comfortable distance" (2010b, p. 143) and thus develop better emotional regulation skills.

Hypnosis can also support the role of action in changing feelings. When you create an intervention that helps a child distinguish between feelings and actions, you can give the message that feelings exist and matter, but we actively do things (even though we don't feel like it) for many reasons—because it's important to someone else, because it's important to us, or because we have learned from experience that we end up feeling better in the end:

> *I know there are times when you don't feel like walking your dog . . . but you do it . . . because he depends on you to take care of him . . . and you told me those walks make you both feel better. . . . And you know there are times when you don't feel like playing what your friend wants to play . . . but you do it because he's your friend. . . . And I'm sure there are times when your mom doesn't feel like going grocery shopping . . . but you need food so she goes. . . . And there are times when I don't feel like shoveling the driveway . . . but I want to get the car out . . . and I'm afraid if we all just did what we felt like . . . or didn't do what we didn't feel like . . . none of us would*

*do much at all . . . or enjoy the feeling of doing something well
. . . or help someone else . . . or learn what we're good at. . . .*

Compartments and Grief

A relatively small number of bereaved children (5–10%) ultimately develop clinically significant psychiatric problems (Kaplow, Layne, Pynoos, Cohen, & Lieberman, 2012; Melhem, Porta, Shamseddeen, Walker Payne, & Brent, 2011; Dowdney, 2000) although many more children (28–40%) experience adjustment or behavioral problems (Dowdney, 2000). Although research on treatment for bereaved children is lacking, studies by Cohen, Mannarino, and Staron (2006) and Layne et al. (2008) show that factors such as social support, the establishment of normal routines, and the emotional functioning of the parents influence how children recover from the death of a loved one. Younger children may experience symptoms of anxiety, while older children experience bereavement similar in symptoms and course to major depression (Kaplow et al., 2012). A thorough review of the many factors influencing and complicating grief is beyond the scope of this book, but I offer here some ideas for the use of compartments as one experiential approach to dealing with the hard work of grieving.

Grieving children are often overwhelmed by the power of their feelings, including sadness, anger, guilt, and fear. Chances are the adults around them are also dealing with their own grief. In addition to the support of adult caretakers, children benefit from strategies that offer them some containment of their grief, permission to move forward after a loss, and the ability to positively reminisce about the person they have lost (Layne et al., 2008; Kaplow et al., 2012). These interventions must be done gently; the goal is to help children process the emotions in a way that is counter to the overwhelming pain they are often trying to avoid and suppress, while giving them some sense of security and emotional regulation.

With younger children, introduce the idea of compartments concretely by drawing or using blocks or boxes. You can also make a box with masking tape on the floor. Allow the child to step in and out as you talk about emotions, memories, the future, or whatever you're addressing. This helps demonstrate movement in and out of strong feelings and memories, and gives the child permission to take a break.

With older children, I make the suggestion, often informally, that I have some ways to manage and understand their strong feelings and memories while they heal, and that we can experiment with compartments (or whatever term works best). Of course, children can certainly come up with their own compartments once they get the hang of what you're teaching them. Here are some of my favorites.

The Future Compartment

Grieving children often feel that nothing will change in the future, and that the level of pain they currently feel will remain constant. Helping a child to gently imagine a future (age progression) where the intensity of her grief will shift and life can have happy moments again is critical to healing.

The Connection Compartment

Children often avoid people, places, and other things connected to the loss. They may feel alone and disconnected from others who, for example, have not lost a parent or a sibling. They may also feel disconnected from the identity they once had: "I'm no longer a sister. I'm different because I don't have a father anymore" (Kaplow et al., 2012). Helping a child imagine reconnecting to important people and other regular aspects of her life—the soccer team, classmates, other relatives—builds back the social supports so important to moving out of depression.

When one 10-year-old girl who had lost her older brother in a car accident told me that she knew she had to figure this out on her own, I told her we would sit together on one of my couches while we talked about her sadness, and then move together to another chair or couch when she wanted to step away from it. She was in charge, but I was right there, moving with her. We made it a point to change which couch was the "sadness couch" from session to session so we could sit on any of the couches when we were doing other things.

The Memory Compartment

Closely related to the connection compartment is the ability for a child to create a nontraumatic memory of the person they have lost, particularly if the child's experience of the death was traumatic (Layne et al., 2008). The memory compartment can be an imagined place where the child has access to the happy memories of the person. He can also have a compartment for the sad memories, a place to visit where he can have his feelings, talk to the person he lost, and accept the normal aspects of his present sadness. I remind you that the purpose here is to create memories that allow the child to move forward with positive memories of the past, while helping him safely experience and express his feelings of loss in the present (Phillips, 2006). It is not an age regression back to traumatic events.

The Me Compartment

Some children need permission to move forward and reestablish their own identity. Particularly if a parent is grieving, the child may have guilt about any positive experiences or feelings, wanting to be loyal to the pain the parent is experiencing. The child benefits from "a place to go inside where it's okay to be you . . . to have fun and laugh . . . to let yourself feel happy and silly sometimes . . . to know that there are many parts of you . . . and that you can still have a fun part . . . a hopeful part . . . that your sadness will be a part of you, too, but not all of you. . . ."

PUTTING IT ALL TOGETHER: SOCIAL SKILLS AND CONNECTION

Just as there is no single factor that leads a child to become depressed, there is no single factor that guides him out of depression. I wish to end this chapter on depression with a focus on how we can hypnotically support the development of better social skills. I have stressed repeatedly that the ability to have positive relationships, feel competent socially, and solve social conflict is critical for the prevention and relief of depression in children. Recognizing the pervasive impact of poor or positive social connections in a child's life is critical (Barlow, 2001; Katz, Conway, Hammen, Brennan, & Najman, 2011). When a child is depressed, the irritability, withdrawal, and lack of engagement can impact friendships; conversely, a lack of social skills and difficulties connecting with peers can lead to isolation and depression (Katz et al., 2011). Anxiety, too, hinders social connection (often contributing to depression by adolescence). Lankton and Matthews stressed the importance of finding solutions that address the "unique interpersonal interactions in the client's daily life" (2010, p. 211).

As you prioritize your goals, keep the question "How does the current framework impact relationships and what will I offer to improve them?" in the forefront of your thinking. For example, a child with a very rigid approach to rules alienates classmates with his unwillingness to compromise during a kick ball game. A child with a too-flexible interpretation of the rules angers his friends when he changes the rules to compensate for an error.

Research abounds on the specific skills children need to succeed socially. Studies have focused on the importance of impulse control, focus, and emotional regulation, all of which create what is termed socially competent behavior (McKown, Gumbiner, Russo, & Lipton, 2009; Payton et al., 2008; Crick & Dodge, 1994). Add to those the need for flexibility, tolerance of frustration and uncertainty, and the ability to engage versus withdraw and isolate. Interpersonal psychotherapy has been shown to be an effective, short-term treatment for depression in adults and adolescents (Markowitz & Weissman, 2004; Mufson, 2010). When used with teens, this approach focuses on "1) identifying a specific problem area; 2) identifying effective communication and problem-solving techniques for that problem area; and 3) practicing these skills in session prior to using them outside of session in the context of significant relationships" (Mufson, 2010, p. 67).

Michael Yapko's (2009) book *Depression Is Contagious* clearly lays out several detrimental (and depression-sustaining) social patterns and what to do about them. He describes the importance of good boundaries, assessing your own thoughts, and developing realistic expectations of others. My teenage clients and their parents have found this book to be a helpful resource. Multiple social skills books are available for kids of all ages. These books list skills for children to practice, often in very helpful and concrete ways. And of course, you could always just ask the child, "To help you feel better with friends, what do *you* think you need to learn?"

Using hypnosis to build social skills, particularly in anxious and depressed kids, follows the same process we've been discussing all along: identifying a needed skill (or group of skills) and then creating a focused, interesting, and supportive experience that allows a child to consider, imagine, and practice using these skills in social situations. Luke and Anika are great illustrations of how a child's depressed frame impacts social connections, and of how to identify and build social skills using hypnosis and homework.

Eleven-year-old Luke, for example, had a propensity to jump to negative conclusions about other children, activities, or interactions. And he was a ruminator: after school he would go on and on about how horrible his day was and how other kids didn't like him. This is a common social struggle for depressed, isolated children, and unfortunately becomes a self-fulfilling prophecy. Luke would head out for recess and automatically assume (and exude) "no one wants to play with me, and their games are dumb, anyway." Kids learned to steer clear of his grouchiness.

Because he was a champion global thinker (not in a happy way), he needed work on identifying parts. We did some role-playing together, imagining recess with his Awful part in charge, and then with his Yes part helping out. He decided he might need a Maybe part that would let him watch and then decide. We drew the parts on three index cards that he could take to school, with my suggestion that he look at them before recess (or anytime he wanted), imagine what each had to say, and choose the part that would make recess more fun. He decided that he would try them all on different days, a move toward flexibility that I encouraged. We then talked about jobs where people "try things and come to conclusions about them," like food testers, movie critics, toy testers, race car drivers, and so on. "I bet you can do the same with games at recess. You can test them out, and see what you think. Some will be fun; some will be dumb. Some will be fun for a bit, but then might get boring. Some will be great, but the teachers will decide it's too dangerous. The trick is to try things out, then decide."

Luke reluctantly took the cards to school and, not surprisingly, reported back that he tried using the Maybe card, but decided that most of the games were dumb. I acknowledged his willingness to observe and gather data. I told him to keep using the cards, but also wanted him to notice five funny things he saw at recess and report back to me, and I'd do the same in my office for the week. I planted the seed that some people could see funny where no one else did— and he was that kind of person. "While everyone else is mad or complaining, you notice the humor. And you can stand there and smile. That's one of the secrets you keep." This made Luke smile. "You can smile on the playground if you like," I said. "My brother was kind of a serious kid like you, but sometimes he would start smiling. And I'd ask him why. And he'd say, 'Oh, just thinking funny thoughts.' And then we'd both be smiling."

Luke is a work in progress. Temperamentally, he has a few hills to climb. But giving him concrete ways to engage, helping him move away from his globally negative assessments of others, and modeling the simple act of putting a smile on his face led to great improvements socially during his fifth grade year. Did I ever do a formal hypnosis session with him? Not really. But I was always looking for ways to plant seeds, make suggestions, and follow them up with experiences that would shake up that stubborn little frame of his. (And I told his mother to buy him a joke book for Christmas.)

Anika, a thoughtful, introverted 16-year-old, illustrates the importance of addressing several patterns that together contribute to social difficulties and subsequent depression.

I met Anika when she was an 8-year-old with separation anxiety. We used hypnosis to bolster her ability to externalize her worry, talk back to its predictable announcements that she couldn't handle things on her own, and tolerate the normal feelings and thoughts of uncertainty when she started new things, like school or music lessons. She did great with that, but then returned years later as a depressed and socially anxious 14-year-old freshman. Her grades were slipping; sleep was poor; and she reported feeling sad much of the time, mainly about "having no friends."

Anika had always been quiet, but had a group of friends that she felt close to until this year. Per her account, she didn't feel included. She was sure that they were doing things without her, but when she was with them, she felt self-conscious about what to say or how to be funny like they were. She began refusing invitations to go places, isolated herself in her room, and told her mother that she was a loser. Her mother was becoming increasingly frustrated by the day. "She is so negative! I try to point out the positives. She actually has nice friends and they try to include her. She refuses to see that. We have the same conversation over and over. It's just getting worse." Her mother reported that when Anika did hang out with her friends, she looked happy. She was laughing and participating. Anika would either deny her mother's observations or state that it was a fluke and probably wouldn't happen again.

Anika's rumination and cognitive rigidity were clear targets for treatment. She was spending a lot of time thinking and talking about what was wrong, and seemed unable to think or act in a problem-solving way. My goal was to loosen her rigid definition of "being a friend" and help shift her attentional bias away from the negative social cues, a ruminative pattern in socially anxious people (Schmidt, Richey, Buckner, & Timpano, 2009). Anika would review, for example, how many (perceived) negative responses she got to a comment, or how long her friends took to return a text. She perseverated on the thought that she was not able to be a good friend because she was too quiet for this outgoing group.

Below are three frames I wanted to introduce in order to move Anika out of her rigid and depressing thought spinning. As you read each of them, take a moment or two to think about how you might convey them to her, and consider other frames that might be helpful as well.

1. There are many different kinds of friends and relationships (to counter Anika's ruminative question, "Why can't I be outgoing like the other girls?").

> Not everyone has to be center stage . . . in fact, the funny guy needs a straight man . . . and the lead singer depends on the band and backup singers. . . . Famous movie stars have their childhood friends that provide an escape from the glitz . . . and a chance to just be who they are on the inside. . . . There are so many different ways to connect and be a solid friend. . . . Maybe you're the loyal one, the steady one, the planner that organizes behind the scenes . . . but doesn't have to be the star. . . . There's value in being quiet . . . observing . . . like the Scottish proverb . . . "Listen twice before you speak once" . . . which you already know so well. . . . Perhaps you can recall

times when that's already helped you manage the drama of
your friends . . . times when you've listened . . . or waited and
watched . . . and then knew better what to do next. . . . Some-
one has to write the stories about your friends, and it's almost
always not the center of attention who does so. . . .

2. When you focus on the negative aspects of an experience, you miss out on the possible positives (to counter her overanalysis of everything she did wrong when with her friends and her ruminative inability to change her focus).

A friend of mine just returned from a vacation to a beauti-
ful island . . . and she was disappointed with the food. . . .
It really was not good . . . and as she talked to me about the
lousy breakfast . . . and the miserable lunch . . . and the so-so
dinner . . . I wondered if she saw any sunsets . . . or what the
beaches were like . . . and if she enjoyed the time with her
family . . . but she never talked about that during our conver-
sation . . . so I wonder what she noticed between meals when
she was there. . . .

3. You will learn by doing (to counter her tendency toward passive and repetitive thinking).

And I know you're in the process of getting your driver's license
. . . and the hours of practice you need . . . and it made sense
when you told me . . . how the time spent in the classroom at
driver's ed . . . pales in comparison to the time spent on the
road. . . . A surgeon I know told me about a phrase they use in
medical training when they're learning to operate . . . "See one,
do one, teach one." . . . They take action . . . in order to learn
. . . and the surgeon laughed when I asked her if there's a time
when they get to think about one for a really long time. . . .

The message that depression is a permanent, defining condition is all too pervasive. I hear more and more parents and children use the language of passivity and resignation when they talk about depression—an unfortunate acceptance of something that they have perhaps been conditioned to see as unchangeable and all too biological. I hope this chapter inspires you to actively go after such seeming permanence, using creative hypnotic interventions to show children and their families the many ways they can become involved in creating an active, connected, enjoyable future. As you will see in Chapter 8, the overlaps continue as we focus on helping children flexibly and actively deal with the emotional and physical aspects of pain and illness.

CHAPTER *8*

Addressing the Physical

Pain, Illness, and
Medical Procedures

*E*llie is an 11-year-old girl undergoing treatment for cancer. She is smart, funny, and spunky, and her prognosis is excellent. Ellie has had to endure significant unpleasantness, not only because of the chemotherapy and all that entails, but because her separated parents have a difficult relationship. Their conflicts are being played out, often loudly, literally at her bedside. Ellie has been vomiting, an expected side effect of the treatment. But the medical team reports that she is vomiting well before they administer the chemo (a common occurrence) and that her anxiety is high.

When I meet with Ellie in my office between treatments, she tells me that her dad has only been coming to the hospital sporadically to visit her. (She's in and out depending on her status.) During his last visit, she says, he talked little and only stayed for a few minutes. Mom, anxious herself and emotionally unpredictable, frequently talks to Ellie about how poorly her father handles things. The boundaries in this family are lousy. Ellie often says her parents are acting "like children." She sighs heavily and tells me, "I just want to get away from this."

So here we have a girl, undergoing chemotherapy, feeling lousy, trapped at times in her hospital bed between her parents' conflict and stress. Of course she wants to get away from this. And I agree. "Let's go!" We've done this before, so she sits back and closes her eyes, and off she goes to the beautiful sailboat she dreams of owning one day. Catching the wind and speeding along the waves, she leaves her cancer, her parents, and her nausea back in New England.

And while she flies, I say to her:

You have learned that you can handle a lot . . . procedures and medications and unpleasantness . . . and you get through it, don't you? You've had to handle dealing with parents . . . and you've even worked on talking to your dad about what you need from him and what you don't . . . with such maturity . . . so while you sail . . . feeling the breeze . . . you can really see . . . from way out there . . . how determined you've been in so many ways. . . . But everybody needs a break sometimes . . . to know when enough is enough . . . and so you've learned how to treat yourself to some alone time . . . some healing . . . some freedom . . . to just go somewhere far away . . . to enjoy being a girl . . . separate from the upset . . . and connected to the peacefulness . . . separate from the noisy battles . . . so your body can focus on the positive battle . . . and knowing how to do that . . . how to focus on your healing . . . well, that's truly a sign of good health . . . you really can sail above it all. . . .

In contrast to the rather barren landscape of literature on the use of hypnosis with depressed and anxious children, information and research abounds on the effectiveness of hypnosis with children in a medical context (see Kohen & Olness, 2011, for a comprehensive overview). As a therapist and anxiety specialist, this distinction between the physical and the psychological in children is an interesting one, but ultimately is perhaps what wordsmiths would call a distinction without a difference.

If you work with children with physical or medical issues, you know that you're treating much more than physical symptoms; in fact, successful outcomes most certainly require significant attention to the biological, emotional, social, and psychological issues of both the child and the worried parents. Separating out the physical and psychological applications of hypnosis with children is necessary to organize research and chapters in books, but I like to believe that those in the world of pediatric hypnosis are most deeply appreciative of the connection between mind and body, between physical symptom and emotional state. When helping a frightened child in pain, the distinctions become less clear and more of an artifice.

In their book *Hypnosis in the Relief of Pain*, Ernest and Josephine Hilgard described the quest to define "pain" and concluded, "We shall find repeatedly that the subjective aspects of pain are paramount in understanding it" (Hilgard & Hilgard, 1975, p. 29). Covino and Pinnell point out that "most medical conditions are neither all physical nor all psychological" (2010, p. 552) and describe the interplay between biological, social, emotional, and cognitive aspects of experience. For example, Szigethy and colleagues (2014) reported depression rates of 25% in youths with inflammatory bowel disease.

Therefore, whether dealing with the acute problem of a broken bone or cut needing sutures, the chronic struggles of conditions like migraines or asthma, or routine procedures like immunizations or dental fillings, introducing families to hypnosis not only paves the way for more positive medical procedures in the future but also teaches a skill that is generalizable to other life circumstances (Kohen, 1986; Calipel, Lucas-Polomeni, Wodey, & Ecoffey, 2005;

Iserson, 2014). Kohen's (2010) long-term follow-up of children treated for headaches with self-hypnosis found that, 9 to 20 years after treatment, 85% reported continued relief from hypnosis, and 50% described the value of self-hypnosis in dealing with life stressors.

When it comes to pain and illness, here's the message I want kids to retain: "Pain" can encompass all sorts of things, and it can be made better and worse by all sorts of things, too. Illness, pain, and stress need not be viewed through separate physical or emotional lenses; they are interwoven and equally valid parts of healing (Phillips, 2006). Hypnosis gives kids and providers a creative tool (as discussed in this chapter) that may be introduced in the context of pain or illness (as with Ellie above), but generalizes to the development of mastery, autonomy, connection, and optimism.

For the purposes of organization (I warned you) I break up the chapter into the categories of chronic pain and illness, acute pain, and medical procedures and surgery. I'll continue to highlight the main therapeutic targets and new frames as a way to further structure your learning. Overlaps are inevitable, although there are certainly some helpful distinctions to be made (for example, acute pain requires a very short induction and immediate suggestions while chronic pain may benefit from more deepening). Your job is to create the intervention that fits Annie or Jacob or Devon, not Headache or Asthma or Chemotherapy.

COPING WITH CHRONIC PAIN OR ILLNESS

Two important points to make at the outset: First, as a psychotherapist, I am not in any way qualified to assess the source of pain or other physical illnesses in a child. I welcome and require a full medical evaluation to identify or rule out medical issues, and see my role as part of a comprehensive medical plan (Elkins, Johnson, & Fisher, 2012). Because I live in the world of childhood anxiety, I often see children with physical symptoms such as headaches and gastrointestinal issues. Their physicians are often fairly confident (based on their evaluation and the child's history) that the source of symptoms is anxiety, but ruling out other possibilities is an important place to start.

Second, it has been my experience that, when treating a child in pain, there is no need (nor ability) for me to define the pain as anything but real to the child. If you've ever had a tension-related migraine, you know it is not a "pretend" headache. The pain you feel and the interruption in your functioning is no less real even when you know the catalyst of the migraine is stress. The goal is to help the child reduce or eliminate the suffering, and when possible resume the normal activities of childhood. How a child comes to perceive, respond, recover, or adapt to pain is the goal of treatment. It's about her understanding of the pain, not yours. Start where she is.

Making concrete statements about the prevalence and precipitants of chronic pain in children and adolescents is difficult because of the varying reports from multiple studies. For our purposes, here are the most consistent conclusions about kids and pain, based on large systematic reviews (Goodman & McGrath, 1991; Roth-Isigkeit, Thyen, Stoven, Schwarzenberger, & Schmucker, 2005; King et al., 2011; Swain et al., 2014):

- Chronic pain in children (defined in many ways but generally reported as at least monthly occurrences for at least 6 months) is common and getting worse.
- Girls report more pain than boys, and reports of pain increase as children age.
- Headaches and stomachaches are the most commonly reported.
- Chronic pain in children impacts multiple levels of functioning and is a likely predictor of chronic pain in adulthood.

Because chronic pain and illness impact children and parents in so many different ways, interventions must be creative and multifaceted. Lonnie Zeltzer, in her book for parents *Conquering Your Child's Pain: A Pediatrician's Guide for Reclaiming a Normal Childhood*, said it well: "By the time the pain has become chronic, it has multiple factors that keep it going, add to its strength, and contribute to functional disability associated with pain. Pain takes on baggage as it gains strength—to stop it, all baggage must be identified, disentangled, and dismantled" (Zeltzer & Blackett Schlank, 2005, p. 11). Her plan includes reducing a child's central nervous system arousal and helping the body heal; supporting the child's return to normal functioning; helping the family cope with the situation; and developing a sense of optimism and even humor in the face of pain.

Pain is complex, subjective, and personal. But it is the very subjectivity of experience that makes hypnosis a valuable asset to a suffering family. Let's talk about interventions that modify a child's relationship to her pain or illness by introducing (1) malleability or variability in expectations, sensations, and perceptions; (2) the use of parts to compartmentalize, dissociate, and discriminate, and (3) a return to activity and engagement in daily life. All aspects of your interactions should move the child toward the broader goal of teaching self-regulation and involvement in managing the many layers of discomfort (Sugarman, 2013; Kohen & Olness, 2011).

Two Frames in One:
Experience Is Variable and the Value of Parts

Children who have been dealing with their pain or illness for a period of time have likely endured significant medical treatment, and may have little reason to trust that you have anything new to offer. Hope is a dangerous stance to take. The emotional risks are high. Imagine that you've been dealing with pain or illness for a long time. Perhaps doctors have told you there's nothing causing the pain, or they know the cause but can't fix it. You may have heard adults talk about your illness as chronic, which to you means it's not going away. Now, you say to yourself, this therapist is going to make things better? Maybe she thinks it's not that bad. Even worse, maybe she thinks it's all in your head. She's not hearing you. She doesn't understand that this is big and bad and real. Rigidity, like a turtle shell, is protective.

You must offer something new, and rapport and positive expectancy are essential. You must quickly connect to the child on multiple levels: acknowledging the reality of the current situation, conveying positive expectations that the child's circumstances can improve, and providing experiences that shake up the physical and emotional patterns. In describing the cycle of negative expectancy and recurrent pain, Sugarman observed that "a critical piece of any hypnotic strategy that hopes to change this negative expectancy is helping a young person have the courage to imagine it can be different" (2013, p. 464). Certainly the same can be said of the depressed, anxious, or grieving child.

On the flip side, there are children who, for whatever reason, have high expectations of what you can do. Perhaps they've heard of hypnosis, or someone has raved about the work you do. Perhaps they see you as their last hope, or by nature they are optimistic and open. The pace with these children may be faster and the energy higher. Take full advantage of this windfall when you come across it.

However the child arrives at your door, the message is packaged accordingly and conveys: "I have something interesting to offer, something different, and I am going to teach you what I know."

To introduce the frame of variability, you must aim to:

- Change the relationship, perception, and meaning of the pain or symptoms by using imagination, surprise, humor, metaphor, and so on
- Teach skills that alter physical sensations
- Increase mastery with ongoing use of the skills

Hypnosis for chronic illness or pain can—and should—target both physical sensations and the emotional correlates. Pain has a variety of meanings to children (Kohen & Olness, 2011), and the emotional and cognitive relationships to chronic pain and illnesses such as asthma, functional abdominal pain, and headaches in children are well documented (see, e.g., Kozyrskyj et al., 2008; Sandberg et al., 2000; Ritz, 2012; Drake & Ginsburg, 2012a; Baumann, 2002). Interestingly, Jensen et al. (2006) showed that hypnosis was beneficial even when the actual pain ratings did not decrease. Subjective rating of pain may have stayed the same, but the sense of well-being increased and stress decreased.

Based on a review of the research on hypnosis and pain management, Feldman proposed that "hypnotic approaches that focus on the affective dimension of the pain may be more effective with more people than the traditional approach that emphasizes relaxation and dissociation from the sensation of pain" (2009, p. 243). Kohen and Olness (2011) wrote that hypnoanalgesia is likely to fail if the emotional dimensions of the pain are ignored. The focus, particularly at the beginning, should be on building momentum with sensory modification versus symptom elimination (Patterson, Jensen, & Montgomery, 2010) because it's both easier for most kids to accomplish and less likely to kick up a child's defenses (Sugarman, 2013). I use a child with chronic headaches as the example here, but please know that the following is not a headache intervention or script.

Preinduction Interview

As you begin the interaction, remember that a hurting child is likely focused on her pain or symptoms, as are the adults around her. Be brief (as you have gathered all the medical history from the adults separately) and ask questions that will give you a picture of how the symptoms look and feel to the child. Ask her to give you words, show you with her hands, or draw a picture of her headache. Listen and watch carefully, as her current perceptions will inform your future suggestions (Kohen & Olness, 2011).

I urge you to be surprising here—don't ask the same old questions. Start demonstrating that this is different from what she's used to. Step away from expected questions and patterned responses. Your questions must also imply disconnection from the pain. How will you immediately begin to dissociate her from her symptoms?

If it were a color, what color would it be? What animal would it be? What does it say to you? Does it have a favorite TV show? Is there anything else about it that you want me to know?

Then ask her what it's like in her head when the discomfort is not there.

When you notice the headache is gone, what color is that? When does that happen? How does that happen? Is there any way you can show me with your face or your hands or your body what you look like when it's gone? Where in the universe are headaches not allowed?

Induction

Introduce the idea of new patterns formally or informally by acknowledging how much attention the headaches demand and how she's had to answer so many questions about them. Let her know how well she was able to tell you (or show you) how they sometimes stay the same but sometimes change, and how you noticed the creative ways she talked about them. I often say (with obvious delight and appreciation), "I've never heard anyone describe it just that way. . . . That's a new way of looking at it. . . ."

Your induction continues with an invitation to notice or do something differently, moving outside of the usual pattern, taking a break:

*And as you sit here now, I wonder if you'd like to learn some
other new things . . . and how to play around with what you
notice . . . play around with what you feel or see or hear. . . .
We all notice different things . . . and can sometimes notice
nothing at all. . . .*

You may choose from any of the induction ideas from Chapter
4, such as an eye fixation or cues to imagine watching images on
a screen. Your choice, however, should portend a focus on change,
adjustments, or altered perception of the symptoms, so pick
accordingly.

Here are some examples (moving from younger to older). The
first example, geared toward young children, combines the induction
and the response set.

*I wonder if we can imagine our hands feeling very warm, like
we were putting them into a nice, warm tub of water . . . yes,
like that. . . . Let's pretend . . . and now let's take them out
and make some snowballs with our bare hands . . . packing
the snow together . . . imagining how that feels . . . freezing!
. . . And now let's pretend we are taking some sips of hot soup
or hot chocolate . . . blowing on it . . . tiny sips . . . and now
we are drinking a cold glass of water . . . with ice cubes . . . so
chilly! We can imagine so many things . . . and make our body
feel so many different ways. . . .*

*Let's see if we can slow down our breathing together . . . nice slow
breaths. . . . Now let's speed them up a bit . . . like your dog pant-
ing on a hot day. . . . Now slow again. . . . See how you can change
the way you breathe? . . .*

*Would you like to see if you can pretend to be heavy like a rock?
. . . Can we pretend that our feet are getting so heavy . . . like they*

are made ot bricks or rocks . . . or your hands are heavy . . . so
heavy you don't even want to lift up your fingers [see Heavy Hands,
Chapter 5] . . . or would you like to feel lighter . . . so that you don't
even feel the chair underneath you . . . lifting up? . . .

As you're sitting here, you can take a few moments to readjust
. . . to move around in the chair . . . to just notice the shifts that
happen . . . when we play around with things . . . when we ease
up with our breathing . . . our blinking . . . the muscles in our
face . . . when we change in some way. . . .

Whatever you choose, help the child experience changes and variations—however small—in her body. Kay Thompson described having her patients tense up their muscles as much as possible, and then notice the warmth, the rush of circulation, and the feeling of lethargy as they let go. She wrote, "When you take some simple physiological steps that you know will work and bring them to the attention of the patient, then you have started to build the foundation of trust you need" (Kane & Olness, 2004, p. 319).

Some tips: Earlier I reminded you to pay attention to the words used to describe the symptoms or pain. Your inductions (and your suggestions) should contrast with the symptom description, not reinforce it. For example, if a child describes his headache as a "heavy throbbing," then don't suggest he make his hands or feet heavy as a way to introduce variability of experience. Instead, ask if he'd like to pretend that his hands are light and floating, or creatively embed suggestions for lightness, such as, "I know you've been dealing with this problem. . . . It's been weighing on you. . . . I think you might like a way to lighten your mood . . . lift your spirits. . . ."

Progressive relaxation is often used as both the induction and initial intervention in medical settings. This approach can help a child calm down his nervous system, decrease arousal, and give him a concrete process to feel loose and relaxed on his own.

However, I caution you to be aware of the length and content of this type of induction and intervention. Younger children, even those not in pain, are unable to maintain focus for long (and even teens and adults may find it boring). More importantly, doing a protracted progressive relaxation exercise may actually replicate the negative trance of focus and vigilance on the body. Be aware, too, that a child has likely heard the instruction to relax from parents or other providers. Has it helped in the past? Then use it. But repeating an instruction that has not worked or that feels predictable as you move from head to toe can create impatience rather than positive expectancy or curiosity about what comes next.

Building a Response Set

Your response set then primes responsiveness to the upcoming suggestions that will ask her to alter both her physical symptoms and her relationship to them. Again, this may be done formally or informally with general statements and descriptions (truisms) that are easy to accept.

First focus on the variety of physical sensations most kids feel:

I've noticed and you've probably noticed how different our bodies can feel . . . from minute to minute or day to day . . . how we go from hungry to full to hungry again . . . from wide awake to tired and sleepy . . . then back to awake . . . or from cold to hot to cold again . . . at the beginning of spring the air feels so warm and we throw off our coats . . . but at the end of summer that same air feels chilly to us. . . . (adapted from Yapko, 2012)

Then emphasize how kids' responses to sensations or experiences vary widely:

> *And it's interesting how sometimes what we feel in our bodies is connected to where we are . . . or what we're doing . . . or what we're feeling . . . how you might forget to feel the scrape on your knee if you're winning the game. . . . But it's not so easy when you're feeling the sting of a loss . . . or how a baby's boo boo gets better when Mom is there to kiss it . . . or sometimes gets worse if Mom looks scared. . . . What a curious mixture . . . of how we feel about how we feel. . . . It's a funny thing . . . to me, at least. . . .*

And continue to build responsiveness toward the concept of parts—dissociation, compartmentalization, and discrimination:

> *We all have our own thoughts and feelings . . . what we find interesting and what we find boring . . . what we pay attention to and what we ignore . . . what we remember and what we forget . . . who knows what will grab your attention next . . . or what will feel big or small. . . .*

Interventions and Suggestions

The groundwork has been laid: we want to shift sensations and affective and cognitive reactions. We want a child to feel better physically—and have more control and confidence emotionally and cognitively. In sum, we want children to feel competent and equipped to address their physical symptoms. Using a variety of ages and presenting issues as content, the following are some examples to spark your creativity as you create variability and preach the value of parts.

Shifting Attention to and Amplifying Nonsymptomatic Parts (Physical and Otherwise)

As you close your eyes and sit back for a few minutes, I wonder if you can find a part of you that feels really good right now . . . maybe it's a part that often feels pleasant . . . or a part you haven't visited with for a bit . . . the wheel that's not squeaky . . . but rolls along. . . . And I don't know what part that is . . . a toe . . . a fingernail . . . your right earlobe or your left elbow. . . . You can nod or tell me when you've said hello to that part. . . . I wonder how you can really welcome that part in . . . or maybe that part should welcome you back. . . . Hey, says your big toe, it's about time we hang out together. . . . You can wonder what you'll do . . . with that pleasant part of you . . . and how you and your toe might enjoy the best parts of you . . . your humor . . . your smarts . . . your energy. . . .

Activating Imagination, Problem Solving, and Mastery

I see you brought your stuffed bear with you. . . . Thank you for doing that . . . because I have a favor to ask of that bear. . . . You told me how you and your bear pretend together and how you two talk and he tells you stories and cuddles with you at night as you fall asleep and goes with you in the car. Such a good friend to have. I wonder if we can ask the bear to pretend something with us. . . . It's not something all bears will do . . . but do you think your bear will help? I'm wondering how your bear can help with your breathing. . . . He helps you a lot, doesn't he? He makes you smile and keeps you company. . . . He looks so cozy sitting there with you. . . . Can we ask him? Maybe the three of us can come up with some ideas together. He knows you much better than I do.

Compartmentalizing, Changing Emotional Response, Use of Humor

I have told this story often to school-age kids and teens.

I had a mailman named Frank. . . . He retired a few years ago. . . . Frank got a lot of attention in the neighborhood . . . but not because of the mail . . . but because Frank wanted to talk and complain. . . . He'd go on and on and on if you let him . . . just stop you in your tracks. . . . Of course the neighborhood needed Frank to do his job . . . and he was very good at delivering the mail. . . . It was the extra stuff we weren't so thrilled about . . . so we figured out ways to handle Frank. . . . Some people just avoided him because his schedule was rather predictable. . . . Some learned to hear the postal truck coming . . . heard the warning in the distance. . . . Some people said a quick hello and announced they had somewhere else to be . . . and some-times Frank would get your attention . . . and talk for too long . . . usually complaining about the same things . . . nothing new . . . and when that happened to me, I'd nod politely for a bit . . . and think about other things that needed my attention . . . might let my mind wander a bit. . . . I knew he was talking but I didn't really listen. . . . One neighbor saw another neighbor caught by Frank . . . so she called the neighbor's cell phone . . . and helped him get away from Frank . . . and they found it funny . . . which became a good strat-egy . . . to keep it light . . . and let Frank move on down the road . . . which he finally did when he retired. . . . And you might wonder what Frank has to do with you . . . or maybe you already know . . . so you can tell me what you're thinking . . . [preparing for the check-in] and I'll tell you why I wanted you to hear about Frank. . . . Frank the mail-man would be happy to know he had a part in delivering such an important message. . . .

Leave Your Pain, Conflict, and Stress
and Go Away (Like Ellie)

*It sounds like you need a break from all of this . . . your head-
aches and your brothers and your schoolwork. . . . That's the
great thing about having an imagination like yours. . . . You can
go away . . . pick a place . . . a real place or an imagined place
. . . and let yourself get absorbed in what you see . . . what you
hear . . . and maybe you're doing something you love to do . . .
or maybe you're just relaxing . . . or maybe you're relaxing here
and doing what you love there. . . .*

Personifying and Modifying the Symptom

Having children personify their pain (or anxiety or depression)
through drawing, description, clay, or role-playing is a common way
to help them get some distance from it, and then change the symptom and their relationship to it. Eight-year-old Garrett, who was
dealing with functional abdominal pain, chose to make his pain
incompatible with his relaxation routine (although he didn't put it
quite that way):

> *My stomachache is a block of ice with sharp edges. Not
> smooth like an ice cube. Like the ice chunks on the side of
> the road. So when I practice my relaxing, I put a heating pad
> on my tummy, and I imagine that the heat just melts the ice. It
> gets smaller and smaller. The heat feels good, too. Then when
> I finish relaxing I go pee, and I'm peeing out the stomachache
> and flushing it down the toilet.*

Brilliant! Garrett and I then practiced imagining having the heating
pad on his tummy when he needed it (usually when he was anxious
at school), so that he could still melt the ice when he wasn't at home
with his heating pad.

Kay Thompson described telling her patients "how pain is really kind of funny. . . . I talk to them about how pain is kind of like a hysterical child and how when it gets started it doesn't know it is safe to stop. . . . What we are doing here is teaching it that it is now safe to stop" (Kane & Olness, 2004, p. 319). This gets a child's attention, and conveys the message that the pain has served its purpose; its message has been received, so it's okay to modify the symptom and the reaction.

Changing the Path of the Pain, or Pain as a Predictable Habit

Paths can be helpful. . . . Deer make paths through the forest and farmers make paths from the farmhouse to the barn . . . and our brains make paths, too. . . . So we don't have to think about every step along the way . . . so when you brush your teeth or do your math facts . . . you can follow that helpful path in your brain. . . . But sometimes brains get stuck on paths that aren't so helpful . . . or we follow a path even when it doesn't take us where we want to go. . . . Milton Erickson was a very clever man who enjoyed the ways of the brain . . . and liked to discover new ways to solve problems . . . and was a master at pointing people toward new paths. . . . He also knew that people would follow paths . . . some that helped and some that didn't. . . . He told a story about how when he was a kid . . . because even as a kid he was learning about making paths and patterns of the brain . . . he would make a crooked path in the snow on the way to school . . . and then would enjoy seeing later how people followed the crooked path even when the road was straight. . . . Sometimes we follow paths . . . automatically. . . . Keep following the steps . . . until you discover a different path. . . .

This can lead into suggestions and skills that change the pattern and encourage new pathways and helpful connections. A child with asthma, for example, can notice the first signs of wheezing and respond by allowing the breathing muscles to relax while the bigger muscles around them relax as well (Kohen, 1986). Because we know the connection between asthma and emotional distress (Anbar, 2003; Sandberg et al., 2000), helping a child understand and connect a physical response to emotional regulation is powerful.

> *When you first feel [problem], you can notice it . . . and take a different first step . . . or second step . . . or maybe a step back. . . . And just letting everything slow down for a minute . . . and letting yourself open up . . . and loosen up . . . your breath, your thoughts . . . your muscles . . . giving yourself a moment to see what can be different . . . and like you've practiced. . . . Here's the way you make a different pathway in your brain . . . in your body . . . no rush. . . . Go inside and look around. . . . You get a say in what happens next . . . what steps you want to take. . . . Let's imagine what you can do. . . .*

Disconnecting From Needing to
Figure It Out or Work on It

Erickson and colleagues (1976) described the hypnotic experience itself as an opportunity to enjoy just being, without having to do anything or know anything.

For some kids with chronic pain or illness, permission to just let the symptom be there, without searching for its source or meaning (assuming this is medically indicated) is a great relief, both in the course of a session and in their lives.

Particularly with symptoms that are anxiety related, spending time analyzing why the symptoms are there or trying to eliminate them altogether tends to escalate the problem. Being okay with the symptoms being there (which often paradoxically results in them not being there) releases children and parents from the consuming patterns of anticipation, questioning, and vigilance.

226

Here's an excerpt from a session with 11-year-old Perry adapted from Erickson's theme of not doing and not knowing. Perry was referred to me because of his frequent vomiting. He had been through many tests and seen many doctors. No physical cause was found, and happily Perry's vomiting improved dramatically with psychotherapy. My interventions were generally conversational and informal. Perry enjoyed coming to see me, and looked forward to making our recordings together.

Let's sit back and take a break together, Perry. We get to do a bit of nothing for a while. No questions, no answers. No knowing. That's okay. This isn't school or a doctor's office. We don't have to know why you throw up. I don't know why it happens. I have some guesses and you have some guesses. Sometimes it's because of what you think. Sometimes it's what you eat. Sometimes it's because you run around too fast. Who knows? Maybe it's something we don't have to fix. Maybe it will happen sometimes, and all the other times it won't. One time I went on vacation and while I was gone I hired some guys to come to my house and fix my floor. It was great. I didn't have to do it! Sometimes at night you go to sleep and you grow. It just happens. You don't have to do it. Your body knows what to do. Maybe the part of your brain that wants to fix things and thinks about things can tell the other part . . . you know, the part that just grows your hair and your toenails and even reads now without even thinking . . . maybe one part can tell the other part to figure it out, and you can just go on being a kid that might throw up sometimes, but won't be throwing up those other times, while your brain parts talk to each other and figure it out.

Suggestions for Hypnoanalgesia and Hypnoanesthesia

There are two types of pain-relieving drugs—analgesics and anesthetics. Analgesia is the relief of pain without total loss of feeling or muscle movement.

Anesthesia is blockage of all feeling, including pain. A child in pain doesn't usually care about the use of the terms hypnoanalgesia or hypnoanesthesia. Finding the images and suggestions that work for the individual child is what counts.

Direct or indirect suggestions that help a child alter the messages between the brain and body have been used for decades. A common image is that of the switchbox, where children create images of the brain as the control center with switches that can turn messages on and off, make them smaller, or alter them. Drawing pictures of the brain, nerves, and body parts is helpful for some children. How they then decide to send and receive messages becomes creative and playful, again changing the emotional atmosphere. One child I worked with imagined her body as a big department store, and she could shut down certain departments by turning off the lights and sending the sales staff home.

Some children respond well to suggestions for numbness, although I use this strategy infrequently when dealing with chronic pain or illness, and find it more applicable when dealing with acute and procedural pain. I offer more details and examples about these techniques in the upcoming sections.

Posthypnotic Suggestions

By now I expect that you have a good idea about how to connect your hypnotic interactions with children to their outside experiences. The important pieces to include:

- A connection to specific situations or more general applications as needed
- A suggestion for ongoing practice
- A positive expectation that ongoing opportunities to use the skills will increase skill, confidence, and automaticity

*There may be many things that remind you of this experience
. . . listening to the recording, of course, or when you begin to
notice a sensation, or when you [fill in the specifics of a child's
routine or triggering experiences that you may have discussed
ahead of time] . . . and you can find yourself doing what you've
learned to do here . . . out there [add specifics as needed] . . .
taking it a step at time . . . remembering how practice helps
create those new paths . . . those different reactions. . . . And
you may even look forward to the chance to see and feel what
you've discovered . . . how much you've learned . . . and how
you'll do what works for you . . . sometimes automatically . . .
without even knowing you're doing it . . . until later. . . .*

Action Counts

A few years ago I hurt my back. Nothing too serious, but it curtailed
my activities significantly while I rehabilitated. After several months,
I was ready to go back to the gym where a group of us work out with
a skilled trainer. After watching me ease my way back in for a week
or two, the trainer said, "Hey, stop moving like someone with a bad
back. Move like you." This stopped me in my tracks. He was right.
I was talking, walking, and moving like someone with a bad back
even though I consciously knew I was better. His statement snapped
me out of the negative "back injury trance" I had been in for months.
It was time to move on from my injury and let it retreat from my
constant awareness.

Children who deal with chronic pain and illness are often stuck
in their own negative trance of fear and avoidance, hesitant to engage
in life's activities (Patterson et al., 2010). Anticipation of what might
happen if symptoms occur ("What if I get a migraine while I'm at the
school dance!") without the confidence to handle what happens is
the same cognitive pattern that keeps panic sufferers in their homes
and anxious children out of school. In fact, because the connection

between chronic pediatric conditions (such as asthma and head-aches) and anxiety is so well established, programs to help parents address their reinforcement of the sick role and its avoidant patterns have been developed and implemented with success (Drake & Ginsburg, 2012a). The strategies described in Chapter 6 are very applicable to this issue as well.

The action counts frame directly addresses the need to increase pleasurable activity, engage in relationships, and step into normal developmental challenges. Combined with all of the interventions described above—the ability to manage, transform, or dissociate from symptoms—taking such actions reinforces the suggestion that "you are more than your illness" and sets out to prove it.

This frame can be the theme of a stand-alone session or incorporated with the others. The emphasis is on reconnecting the child with what he can do separate from his symptoms or illness.

With older kids and teens, I mainly rely on a two-pronged approach to first build confidence in the ability to move forward in the face of challenges (physical and emotional), and then some mental rehearsal to create positive anticipation and expectancy. Younger children do well with mental rehearsal, creating a story about what they like to do, and role-playing favorite activities. For example:

> *You have learned so many things about how to manage your [problem]. You can take a few moments right now to think about what you're doing to help yourself . . . the way you practice your breathing . . . and how you so creatively decided to [fill in child's strategies] . . . and the goal all along has been to help you be you. . . . You told me when we first met how much you enjoy [activity] and how good you are at [activity] . . . and now on your own . . . you've been learning these new ways of handling your body and brain. . . . You've been making new*

*pathways and changing old habits. . . . Maybe you've already
had some thoughts or ideas about doing stuff you love to do
. . . or maybe right now . . . the ideas can pop up in your
imagination. . . .*

*I like stories about people who come up with ways to get things
done. . . . Sometimes people said it couldn't be done . . .
grownups who told kids to stop dreaming so big . . . because
they might just end up being disappointed . . . but there's a
young guy who climbed all the highest peaks in the world . . .
even though he went blind at thirteen . . . and a boy I knew
who is in a wheelchair . . . and went to train with his new ser-
vice dog . . . in the middle of a hurricane. . . . Do you know
the story of the 4-minute mile? . . . For decades and decades
everyone said running a mile in less than 4 minutes was
impossible. . . . For decades that was considered a fact . . .
until Roger Bannister did it in 1954. . . . His record only lasted
46 days . . . because once he did it . . . I guess others who
watched him believed it was possible. . . . Funny how what we
watch can make us believe. . . .*

*And so I wonder what you can watch yourself do . . . the
things you already know how to do. . . . You can watch yourself on your mind's computer [screen] and remember . . . and
feel the fun or the effort. . . . Maybe you were laughing or concentrating . . . or just playing without even needing to think
about much at all. . . . You can nod your head or tell me about
what you're imagining if you like [check-in] . . . and let's jump
into the future for a bit . . . and see yourself doing what you
told me you love to do [can talk about specifics]. . . . You'll
take with you what you learn here . . . into those activities out
there. . . . Lots of people rehearse what they're going to do . . .
even in a daydreamy way . . . and you can take a few minutes*

to imagine or rehearse inside your own mind . . . or you can talk to me about it, too. . . . Whatever you like. . . . [potential check-in]

You know how I like to give you ideas . . . but you also come up with your own . . . usually better than mine these days. . . . I'm going to remember your ideas . . . and you can remember this idea when you need to . . . the idea of taking action . . . of doing stuff . . . of having fun. . . . Maybe you'll take this idea and run with it . . . or walk with it . . . or jump on it . . . or hop to it. . . .

Finally, Gfeller and Gorassini (2010) wrote of the importance of describing hypnosis for pain as an active process in which subjects should be taught to focus on and engage with the imagery suggested, rather than passively waiting for the suggested numbness or other sensation to occur. Helping children to see hypnosis as a skill that is developed through active practice will increase the effectiveness of your suggestions.

ACUTE PAIN AND INJURY

Before I address acute pain or distress in children, let me reiterate that using hypnosis with children, particularly when a child is suffering or in pain, is by no means separate or distinct from how caring clinicians interact with their patients. In fact, being hypnotic and the use of hypnotic communication during these types of interactions is likely the rule rather than the exception. My intent here is to identify and enhance the strategies that improve such communication, hopefully making the use of hypnosis even more deliberate, more strategic, more effective, and more commonplace. Sadly, there is a lack of training in the use of hypnosis in emergency care despite its proven value as an adjunct to treatment in these settings (Iserson, 2014; Kohen & Olness, 2011; Salazar, Faintuch, Laser, & Lang, 2010; Sugarman, 2013.

In general, the frames, strategies, and goals I've described thus far also pertain to a child who is injured or experiencing acute pain. The clinician must:

- Build rapport, trust, and positive expectancy
- Address the emotional state of the child
- Create experiences of malleability and dissociation, as needed

But all of these must be accomplished in an acute environment, with the different demands of time and intensity. Rapport, induction, and suggestion are virtually simultaneous. Let's talk specifically about how to work within the demands and requirements of this setting.

Unlike a routine doctor's visit or therapy appointment, you as the clinician have less time. Rapport must be established immediately. Lang and colleagues (1999) encourage the development of rapid or instant rapport by matching the verbal and nonverbal communication patterns, responding to requests, and avoiding negative suggestions, such as, "How bad is your pain?" and "This is going to hurt, but you can be brave." Lang and colleagues (2005) also dispel the seemingly sympathetic practice of alerting patients to impending pain ("Now this will burn a bit") and instead teach a focus on words that invoke comfort or disconnection.

Clinicians should convey confidence that they will be able to help but should also give simple suggestions that increase the child's sense of control, important seeding for the participation you will want to elicit in the immediate future:

We know what to do. . . . You and I are going to work together. . . . You are hearing my words . . . and I am hearing your words. . . . I'm here to help . . . but you are the boss of your

> *body. . . . I'm going to teach you some things. . . . That way*
> *you and I can be in charge of our own jobs . . . what we'll each*
> *need to do. . . .*

Or:

> *I'm going to show you something. . . . Lots of kids think it's*
> *cool. . . . You get to do it. . . . I'll help you. . . .*

These situations are frequently intense—emotions run high; perceived consequences loom large; time is of the essence. The child is more vulnerable, and because of this, more suggestible (Patterson et al., 2010; Kohen & Olness, 2011). Attention to your words—and the potential for both positive and negative impact—is paramount. Research and clinical experience emphasize the powerful role of expectancy in the perception of pain. Koyama, McHaffie, Laurienti, and Coghill (2005) used fMRI scans to measure the activation of pain-related regions in the brain and found that positive expectations for decreased pain were comparable to an analgesic dose of morphine.

Inductions should be brief and direct, and should seed the hypnotic strategy that you are going to employ; ongoing suggestions then amplify the experience. Lynn and Kirsch (2006) suggest the use of imagery that targets and isolates the affected area, compared to suggestions for broader relaxation with chronic or more generalized pain. Communication between you and the child should be frequent and may be done verbally or through signaling with finger raises, blinks, or, as described below, hand squeezes.

Below are some of my favorite takes on different strategies. As always, let input from the child and your mutual creativity be your guide. And even in serious situations, allow for playfulness and some surprises.

Dissociation by Going to a Different Place

Kate, I want you to look right at my face . . . or you can close your eyes and listen to my voice. . . . I have an invitation for you, like an invitation to a party . . . or an invitation to wherever you most like to go [dissociation]. . . . And while you're there . . . for as long as you want to be there . . . you can let us be here . . . doing our jobs . . . for a minute or two [time distortion]. . . . You'll barely notice. . . . Does that sound okay to you?

. . .

I'm going to hold your hand . . . and very gently squeeze it five times. . . . Our hands will talk to each other . . . send messages back and forth. . . . And while I give your hand five squeezes . . . that is your invitation . . . your message . . . to go somewhere fun in your imagination. . . . Do you know where you'd like to go? Great. . . . Five squeezes . . . and every squeeze is a message to go to the [fun place]. I'll count and you go on ahead . . . and when you get there, squeeze me back. . . . Great. . . . Now you can be there . . . and if you want to tell me anything about your adventure . . . go ahead and squeeze my hand again. . . . Send me another message . . . and my little squeezes will be reminders to have fun where you are. . . .

You can time your little squeezes to coincide with medical procedures. Or:

It's funny how you can leave your body here and take your imagination somewhere else . . . like when you daydream during school . . . or dream at night in your bed. . . . Can you go somewhere else? . . . What do you like to do . . . for real or even when you're just pretending? . . . If you want to tell me I can join you there . . . or you can go on your own . . . and nod your head when you get there. . . .

Shifting the Perception of Sensation and Emotion
From Big to Small

You told me you feel scared . . . that you were very scared
when you fell. . . . That's a strong feeling to have. . . . I know
that. . . . There are so many different ways to feel that way . . .
but I'm going to help you let the scared get a bit smaller . . .
shrink it down . . . because with every second that passes
. . . you're more okay. . . . Your heart is finding its way back
to calm. . . . Your breathing is finding its way back to normal.
. . . That's right . . . that sensation of scared can change into
something else. . . . What do you think? Worried? Nervous?
Annoyed? Tired? . . . You can choose whatever you think [e.g.,
child chooses tired]. . . . Yes, sometimes scared turns into tired
. . . because such a strong feeling can tire us out. . . . So with
each breath . . . you can feel the scared getting tired . . . slow-
ing itself down. . . . That's right. . . . Your whole body slowing
down. . . .

Or:

How big do you think the hurt was? [Notice the use of past
tense.] Was it as big as an elephant? Or a moose? Can you pick
an animal that was the size of the hurt? [You can use fruits,
dinosaurs, planets. One child I treated had just studied the
states, so she used Texas as big and worked her way down to
Rhode Island.] . . . Great! Now let's make that animal smaller.
[If possible, child can use hands to show decrease in size as
you model that as well.] . . . Maybe we can change it to a dif-
ferent animal . . . a moose to a chipmunk? Or a whale to a
goldfish? You've made the hurt on your leg so tiny! . . . Now
when we fix it . . . you might not even be able to feel what's
happening. . . . You know it's there . . . but hardly. . . . Things

can go from big to small. . . . Can you think of things that go
from big to small? . . . I was watching a jet in the sky last week
. . . and it kept getting tinier and tinier. . . . I could see the
white line in the sky . . . but then that began to fade, too. . . .
Or a big ice cream cone . . . that keeps getting smaller . . . lick
by lick . . . disappearing!

Creation of Hypnoanesthesia

As described above, direct suggestions for hypnoanesthesia can involve first talking to a child about how the brain receives and sends messages. An acute setting is less amenable to drawing or stories, but I use a simple and direct suggestion for numbness or anesthesia by starting with a description of tuning out:

You told me you have a brother, right? I have a brother, too. . . .
So you must know how to tune out, right? It's like when your
brother or your mom or your teacher says something . . . but
you are interested in something else. . . . So you don't really
hear them. . . . You sort of hear them . . . but not really . . .
just in the background. . . . Has that happened to you? . . . Or
maybe sometimes your mom or dad tunes you out . . . when
they're on the phone or the computer. . . . Well . . . our brains
have a way to tune out lots of things . . . and we can tune out
sounds . . . like noise . . . and body noise, too. . . . Your brain
can tune out messages . . . can shut them off . . . and even
make a part of you numb . . . this part right here. . . . So that
when I touch it . . . or when [medical provider] touches it . . .
it doesn't feel it . . . or it feels like someone else's hand . . .
strange! Let's practice that together. . . .

With older children and teens, you can do a more formal induction, having them close their eyes:

Begin to shift into your imagination, changing your focus from
out to in . . . tuning out what's going on around you. . . . You
tune out the hum of the refrigerator at home . . . or the buzz of
voices in the cafeteria at school . . . or the earrings in your ears
. . . or whatever else you choose . . . at this moment to ignore.
. . . Such a handy skill to have. . . .

You may then ask and draw on common experiences of numbness, such as numb fingers or toes or chins after playing in the snow, a numb lip after a trip to the dentist, or that numbness and tingling we feel when a foot falls asleep.

And that numbness . . . doesn't take much. . . . Your brain is happy
to listen to that type of suggestion . . . something it knows well . . . the
tuning out . . . for a bit. . . .

The glove anesthesia technique is very common, and involves imagining or acting out the placing of a glove of anesthesia (or numbness) onto the hand, creating a hypnoanesthetic, and then transferring the numbness to other parts of the body with the "gloved" hand. I have found numbness to be a more common experience for kids and less medically triggering than the term *anesthetic*, but some children are familiar with topical or local anesthetic from other procedures. It is simply a matter of preference and practice.

Posthypnotic suggestions, often offered in a conversational way, should be used to promote healing and recovery, set expectations for future pain management, and to build confidence and esteem in a general way:

Based on what you did today, I am excited to see how well
you'll heal . . . how you'll help your body . . . by letting it heal.
. . . Now that we're done, I hope you've noticed what I noticed
. . . what we all noticed . . . that you discovered something

really cool . . . the ability to handle a difficult situation . . .
to manage your brain and your body. . . . I don't know when
you'll use these skills again . . . maybe when you come back
to [get sutures removed, have your arm checked, get the cast
removed, etc.] . . . but it's nice to know those skills are inside
of you. . . .

MEDICAL PROCEDURES AND SURGERY PREPARATION: SPECIAL CONSIDERATIONS

Overall, the interventions used with chronic and acute pain are also applicable to children preparing and recovering from surgery and planned medical procedures. For example, children undergoing surgery and cancer treatment will benefit from the ability to:

- Move between connection and disconnection
- Create malleability of experience through sensory alteration or hypnoanesthesia
- Manage the emotional components of the experience
- Develop a sense of mastery

Therefore I won't go through each of the frames again individually, but instead highlight some distinct aspects that are worthy of special attention.

At the top of this list is the relationship between presurgical anticipatory anxiety, general anesthesia, and postoperative recovery. Not surprisingly, presurgical anxiety negatively impacts the procedure and recovery in several ways (Kain, Mayes, Caldwell-Andrews, Karas, & McClain, 2006; Fortier, Del Rosario, Martin, & Kain, 2010; Cohen-Salmon, 2010) and evidence shows that hypnosis can help.

Hypnosis was found to reduce the distress and duration of the procedures, by itself or combined with other treatments such as local anesthetic (e.g., Accardi & Milling, 2009; Tomé-Pires & Miró, 2012; Butler, Symons, Henderson, Shortliffe, & Spiegel, 2005). Liossi and colleagues did a series of studies (Liossi & Hatira, 1999, 2003; Liossi, White, & Hatira, 2009) with children undergoing cancer treatment, and found that the combination of local anesthetic and hypnosis resulted in less anticipatory and procedural anxiety, procedural pain, and behavioral distress.

Zeltzer, Dolgin, LeBaron, and LeBaron (1991) compared hypnosis to nonhypnotic cognitive distraction with pediatric chemotherapy patients and found that the hypnosis group had the greatest reduction in both anticipatory and postchemotherapy nausea and vomiting. Anticipatory nausea and vomiting occur in about 25% of all pediatric cancer patients.

A study by Calipel and colleagues (2005) compared the effect of hypnosis versus the common presurgery medication midazolam on preoperative anxiety and postoperative behavioral problems. Postoperative behavioral disorders include increased separation anxiety, fear, sleep and eating disturbances, and aggression. Symptoms can last for days or weeks after surgery. The children who received hypnosis met the anesthesiologist in their room immediately prior to the surgery. The doctor then established and maintained a "hypnotic relationship" with the child up until the induction of anesthesia. The use of hypnosis compared to the midazolam reduced the reports of behavior disorders by at least half on day 1 and day 7.

Calipel's article is unfortunately vague when describing the hypnotic interventions, but a program designed by Martin and colleagues (2011) identified specific desirable and undesirable adult behaviors impacting anxiety in children during the induction of anesthesia. The helpful behaviors included nonprocedural talk, humor, giving actual control, and a reframing of medical procedures as something fun or positive. The undesirable talk included reassurance and empathy, apologizing, medical talk, and giving implied control (e.g., "Would you like to begin the procedure now?").

Although the authors never used the term *hypnosis*, the use of positive suggestion, reframing of experience, surprise, and development of mastery are obviously modes of positive communication that can be delivered hypnotically (and probably are) in an informal way, enhanced by the focus, attention, and vulnerability of a child in this setting. The authors wrote, "These [desired] behaviors serve to distract children from their emotions and/or help to *reframe a new, potentially frightening environment to something that is manageable and understandable,* such that it is related to lower anxiety levels and increased coping behavior by children" (Martin et al., 2011, p. 20, emphasis added).

Which reminds me of a story about reframing. . . .

Carla, a young woman in her 20s, was seeing me for a chronic medical condition that required numerous medical procedures over a few years. During one session, as she was preparing for an upcoming hospital visit, construction was in full swing in the lot behind my office. We were recording the session, so I knew she heard the constant beeping of the trucks during our session, and would easily hear them again when she practiced later. I began the session this way:

Carla, go ahead and get comfortable . . . in your usual way . . . allowing yourself to focus on letting go . . . settling in . . . and I'm sure we'll both notice as I talk . . . as you listen . . . the beeping of the trucks . . . the revving of their engines . . . even the voices of the workers. . . . Every day I've been hearing this . . . and it makes me smile . . . because I remember a trip I took to an old inn a few years ago . . . and as we sat in the dining room . . . full of atmosphere . . . among antiques and candlelight . . . I kept hearing a beeping . . . the sound of a construction vehicle . . . but it was late at night. . . . Who would be doing construction in the dark? . . . So I asked the waitress. . . . "Oh," she told me, "that's Howard. . . . He's an African grey parrot in the parlor. . . . He's imitating the delivery trucks that back out of the driveway during the day." . . . And so as I hear this construction beeping . . . it reminds me of something else . . . that makes me smile. . . . It brings me to somewhere else. . . .

I continued with the session, amplifying the frame of noticing what we connect to and disconnect from "and how one thing is a reminder of something else . . . in rather unexpected ways . . . transporting you . . . to an enjoyable place in your mind and your memory. . . ."

Carla returned for another appointment about a month after her procedure. "I was in the hospital, and you know how they hook you up to all those monitors? And the beeping just reminded me of the African parrot at the inn . . . and of you telling me that story while I was so relaxed on your couch. . . . Every beep was a little happy reminder."

Helping a child connect to the various procedure-related sounds and sights in a memorable, amusing way interrupts the negative anticipation and shifts the emotional tone. How about anchoring a word that you know will be repeated by the medical staff to a silly joke, image, or even a little bribe?

> *Every time anyone says the word* arm, *you get a point, and for every point, I pay you a piece of bubble gum!*

> *You told me about your favorite memory . . . when you picked up your new puppy Roscoe. . . . Do you remember that? . . . I have an idea. . . . Let's tell the nurse to say the word* Roscoe *. . . or whatever word you like . . . and when she does . . . you can close your eyes . . . bring up that TV screen . . . and watch that memory again. . . . Let's practice it now together. . . . I'll record it and you can listen as much as you like. . . . You can even practice with your mom. . . .*

Hypnotic suggestions can be used formally or informally, as time and setting permit.

Because surgery and cancer treatments are often scheduled, clinicians have more time to prepare the child. (The downside of this is more time for anticipatory anxiety.) Storytelling and modeling with younger children, as always, are effective ways to absorb them and get them to practice. Kohen and Olness (2011) described a 6-year-old boy who benefited from watching a video of another child using hypnosis during a lumbar puncture. Linden (2007) used a doll as a way to communicate, recognizing the usefulness of externalizing a part of the child onto a toy.

A focus on sequencing can be particularly helpful when preparing a child for surgery or a procedure. Dr. Paul Urbanek (personal communication, 2014), a pediatric orthopedist, described the helpful process of having a tour prior to the surgery, where the child can ask questions, see the ward, and visualize what will happen. You can then take this information and create a session with the child that sequentially connects different steps of the procedure to suggestions for coping, mastery, dissociation, or even humor. Dr. Urbanek told me all surgeons are mandated to meet with the patient before the procedure and initial the surgical site with a magic marker. What a great opportunity for some creative seeding and suggesting:

> You'll get to the hospital and go from step to step . . . just like you practiced . . . and you might feel all sorts of things . . . but you know . . . as you go from step to step . . . that Dr. Urbanek will come in to say hello and to sign your arm with his magical marker. . . . You can look forward to that with a little smile . . . waiting for him . . . knowing when he arrives . . . you can take a nice deep breath and feel a little giggle inside . . . or a smile come across your face . . . imagining what silly face you would draw . . . remembering all the silly faces we drew here today . . . and you can take that smile with you. . . .

Posthypnotic suggestions should continue to incorporate the frame of sequencing, with a focus on the steps of recovery. Lobe (2013) listed specific suggestions for recovery to be made in a preoperative session, including relaxing the muscles around the body part where the surgery is occurring, breathing deeply to fill the lungs, a return to normal bowel and bladder function, an appetite after the surgery, and comfort when awakening from the anesthesia. Suggestions for resumed activity (as appropriate) and age progression into the future where healing has occurred and the child is well are also helpful.

Our language reveals that physical and emotional hurts are often woven together, as we suffer from broken hearts, deal with our pain-in-the-neck boss, and shoot ourselves in the foot. As I said earlier, when we teach children hypnotic skills that allow them to manage their illness and pain, their sense of mastery bleeds into other areas, giving them a sense of mastery in dramatic and concrete ways. Although the research on the effectiveness of hypnotic strategies in medical settings is extensive, I have frequently come across the concern that training and delivery are too time consuming and complex. They aren't. Simple metaphors, stories, and suggestions, offered with focus and connection, can make a world of difference. If nothing else, simply reframing language from the negative to the positive should provide a significant step forward.

CHAPTER *9*

Solving Sleep Problems

*N*o one who knew Theo would call him easygoing. The first day of school, a routine visit to the dentist, or a new babysitter resulted in a typical pattern of worrying, crying, and sometimes angry tantrums. At bedtime Theo delayed sleep for hours until his mother finally agreed to sleep with him. His parents had been able to manage (and unknowingly nurture) his demands with consistent doses of accommodation, reassurance, and rearranging of schedules. It was tiring, but they accepted such efforts as necessary to help Theo cope. And generally it worked, as long as everyone played by the rules. But when Theo's chronic difficulty falling asleep worsened at the start of fifth grade, family life became unmanageable. His parents tried their standard approaches, working hard to convince Theo that he could fall asleep: sitting with him, sleeping with him, letting him watch television or play on the computer. They had never sought help before—or even thought that Theo's issues were that unusual—

until Theo announced one night that from now on, if he were awake, the whole family would be awake too. He then proceeded to follow through with his plan. After three sleepless nights for a family of five, his parents called the pediatrician, desperate for help with their family emergency. Everyone was exhausted, angry, and unable to function. The disruption was intense and getting worse by the day. The loss of sleep was the tipping point.

Few family issues garner as much attention as disrupted sleep. The inability to satisfy this most basic of needs is a hot topic among new parents of infants and experienced parents of teens, and many parents in between—and with good reason. An estimated 10–25% of infants, children and teens struggle with some type of sleep disorder. Between 1993 and 2004, approximately 18.6 million visits were made to office-based physicians for sleep-related difficulty in children 17 years of age or less, with the greatest number between ages 6 and 12 (Stojanovski, Rasu, Balkrishnan, & Nahata, 2007). Sleep problems include difficulty transitioning to bed and then falling asleep and maintaining sleep; nightmares, night terrors, and sleep-walking.

In the 12-year period between 1993 and 2004, 81% of children seen by a pediatrician or family physician for a pediatric sleep problem were prescribed a sleep medicine (Stojanovski et al., 2007) and 23% of pediatricians surveyed by Owens, Rosen, and Mindell (2003) reported using medication in otherwise healthy children who had difficulty falling or staying asleep. Yet despite the prevalence of sleep problems in children and the high use of medications, researchers repeatedly report a lack of understanding, treatment options, and training regarding pediatric sleep issues in the medical community (Owens et al., 2003; Owens, Rosen, Mindell, & Kirchner, 2010; Pelayo, Chen, Monzon, & Guilleminault, 2004).

What's going on with kids and sleep? Sleep difficulties appear at first glance to fall into two broad categories: primary problems with sleep (sometimes behavioral, situational, or family related) that result in impaired functioning because of sleep deprivation, and second-ary problems with sleep as a result of other issues, such as illness or pain, anxiety, trauma, or attention-deficit disorder. A lack of sleep is known to negatively impact mood, attentiveness, academic perfor-mance, pain, and even risk-taking behavior in adolescents (O'Brien & Mindell, 2005; Wolfson & Carskadon, 1998). A 4-year study found that children with persistent sleep problems had a 16-fold risk for psychosocial problems, particularly aggression, social and attention problems, and anxious or depressed mood (Simola, Liuk-konen, Pitkäranta, Pirinen, & Aronen, 2014). On the flip side, cer-tain diagnoses such as anxiety, depression, migraine, and ADHD impact sleep, thus making evaluation of sleep patterns an important part of assessment and diagnosis (Alfano, Zakem, Costa, Taylor, & Weems, 2009; Hiller, Lovato, Gradisar, Oliver, & Slater, 2014; Chase & Pincus, 2011; Heng & Wirrell, 2006).

When addressing a child's sleep issues, it can be difficult to know with certainty whether the sleep problem is the cause or the consequence of another childhood diagnosis—or both. Shanahan, Copeland, Angold, Bondy, and Costello (2014) found that sleep prob-lems early in life predicted an increased risk of being diagnosed with generalized anxiety disorder, depression, or oppositional-defiant dis-order later in life. Conversely, generalized anxiety disorder, opposi-tional-defiant disorder, and depression predicted an increase in sleep problems over time. Pressman and Imber's research on sleep issues and ADHD determined that despite a stable 5–6% rate of ADHD in children, 25% of parents reported being told by their doctor that their child should be medicated for ADHD, likely influenced by bed-time concerns: "In the context of our study, we note that there are very strong relationships between bedtime practices/routines and the frequency with which a parent may be advised to consider medica-tions reserved for ADHD in particular" (2011, p. 414). Cassels looked at reactive bed sharing as the result of sleep difficulties (versus inten-tional bed sharing as a parenting choice), and concluded, "the correlates of sleep problems include similar behaviors to those found in ADHD, making false diagnosis not only possible but probable" (2013, p. 14).

Alfano and colleagues (2009) examined the relationship between internalizing disorders in children and teens, and found correlations between anxiety and sleep issues in younger children, while teens with sleep difficulties were more likely to be depressed. They, too, acknowledged the interplay:

> *Although the nature of these data does not allow for conclusions regarding directionality, relationships between sleep and affective functioning seem to be bidirectional. Internalizing problems may give rise to and exacerbate sleep difficulties, while the effects of insufficient sleep include decreased affective regulation and coping skills. . . . Thus, persistent sleep disturbance may contribute to the development of internalizing disorders vis-à-vis an overall reduction in regulatory skills. However, because data are generally limited, experimental and longitudinal research is needed to better understand these complex relationships. (p. 509)*

And it should come as no surprise that family relationships and parenting appear to factor strongly into a child's sleep patterns. Maternal depression and family conflict have been shown to impact a child's ability to fall asleep, perhaps because of increased vigilance and emotional insecurity (El-Sheikh, Kelly, Bagley, & Wetter, 2012). Ng, Dodd, Gamble, and Hudson (2013) found that dysfunctional beliefs about sleep, including a catastrophic view of the consequences of insomnia and a sense of helplessness about the predictability of sleep, are often shared by parent and child, and proposed a possible relationship between the parent's dysfunctional beliefs about sleep and the child's sleep-related problems. Noble, O'Laughlin, and Brubaker (2012) examined sleep problems in children diagnosed with ADHD and found a significant positive correlation between parenting stress and the parent's report of child sleep difficulty, and a significant negative correlation between parenting stress and the implementation of consistent bedtime routines. "Results suggest that a lack of a bedtime routine, in particular, is associated with greater bedtime resistance, which may result in increased parent–child conflict, as well as reduced quality and quantity of child sleep" (Noble et al., 2012, p. 49). They acknowledged that directionality is unknown, but recognized the chicken-and-egg nature of sleep problems, parental stress, and increased affective symptoms.

Untangling all the factors that impact a child's sleep is tricky at best. For our purposes, the relationship between a child's ability to sleep and other problems is most importantly seen as a cycle that spirals downward, as in the case of Theo. Furthermore, the impact of sleep problems appears to be long lasting: sleep difficulties in childhood predict anxiety (Gregory et al., 2005) and depression in adulthood (Touchette et al., 2012). It is reasonable to conclude that addressing a sleep issue directly and early is a smart choice for children and their families (Alfano et al., 2009). Like social connection, the ability to fall asleep and sleep well is a skill that supports children in every area of growth, learning, and self-regulation.

Hypnosis once again may serve as a vehicle to help a child develop the needed skills to sleep better. Multiple reports have described success using hypnosis for sleep-onset problems (Anbar & Slothower, 2006; Graci & Hardie, 2007; Kuttner, 2009) and nightmares and night terrors (Gehrman & Harb, 2011; Kohen, Mahowald, & Rosen, 1992; Kramer, 1989; Taboada, 1975). Levine (1980) and Hawkins and Polemikos (2002) described success with children and insomnia using hypnosis and storytelling. Levine used personalized fairy tales to indirectly introduce coping strategies. Hawkins and Polemikos described a sleeping game where children imagined going to a favorite place and talking to a friendly animal.

A hypnotic experience bolsters the discovery of what works and interrupts the patterns that don't. Like the physical issues discussed in Chapter 8, sleep problems have commonalities and distinctions. With the combination of helpful new frames and behavioral tactics, let's get to work at getting kids to sleep.

EXPERIENCE IS VARIABLE

Edward was an anxious rule follower. He constantly chided his parents and younger sister to stay on time, and fretted each morning about catching the bus, the quality of his homework, and whether or not other children would cause trouble at lunch. Bedtime for him was full of rules and requirements. Lighting, pillow, sounds all had to be just so. "I have schedules in my head all day," he told me. "At bedtime, I lie on one side for a few minutes, then I switch to the other side, then I lie on my back, and I need to fall asleep within 15 minutes or I start to freak out." Almost every night, Edward would watch the clock and miss his self-imposed deadline. His anxiety would escalate, ending in tears, hopelessness, and sleep deprivation. The worry about bedtime was showing up earlier and earlier in the day, and his mood was becoming increasingly depressed.

Edward needed a way to manage sleep (and life) with a little more wiggle room. He needed skills to help him adjust to the variability of sleep, change his rigid, unhelpful beliefs about sleep, and experience variability (namely relaxation) in his body.

Children have difficulty transitioning from waking to sleeping for a variety of reasons, but this first frame of variability focuses most specifically on children who have what we might term sleep performance anxiety. To loosely borrow a line from Franklin Roosevelt, the only thing that keeps these children awake is the fear of staying awake itself. Well, not entirely, but their concerns at bedtime are less about monsters or darkness or kidnappers than about the consequences of not sleeping, beliefs often shared and communicated by their parents (Ng et al., 2013). These children often say, "If I don't fall asleep, I won't do well on my test (or I'll get sick, or play badly in my basketball game, etc.)."

The hypnotic intervention helps to create physical relaxation, but also focuses on normalizing the many ways that kids (healthfully) transition to sleep. Flexibility is the message, as kids that are anxious about the process of falling asleep often believe it is a linear process that should happen in a certain way every night. Because they tend to have little confidence in their ability to put themselves to sleep—and then become trapped by their worries about not being able to fall asleep—they need to hear about the natural variability of the process and learn to challenge, disrupt, and ultimately overthrow their belief that only adherence to rigid rituals will produce the desired outcome.

First: Some Logistics When Doing a Sleep Session

A session designed to help a child fall asleep is a bit different than other sessions, because you actually want the child to fall asleep. If you are conducting and recording the session in your office (as always, I recommend recording sessions whenever possible), it's important to inform the child about the differences and to be permissive about how they'll respond in the office. Some children will not want to fall asleep in your office or won't be able to because of the time of day, in which case I have them sit and "listen" (with eyes closed or open) to relieve any pressure. I make the suggestion that the office is not their bedroom and it's not their bedtime either, so even though they might fall asleep, circumstances will be different at night when they're tired and weary and cozy in their bed.

To introduce a sleep session, I say something like this:

Usually when I make recordings with kids, I want them to stay awake and hear what I have to say, and think their different thoughts. I often ask questions and check in. But this kind of

*recording is a bit different. . . . This is to help you fall asleep,
so you might let yourself drift off and snooze a bit whenever
you like, and I won't interrupt that. At the end of this recording,
I won't ask you to open your eyes—that would be silly! I'll just
say goodnight or sweet dreams . . . or whatever you'd like me
to say. . . . Do you have any ideas about that? [Discuss ideas to
incorporate, then continue.]*

*Today, after I say goodnight [or whatever as been dis-
cussed] on the recording, I'll stop recording, and then I'll tell
you we're done. . . . And if you do fall asleep here (and kids
sometimes do), I'll just wake you up. At home when the recording ends you might be asleep, or on the verge of sleep, or you
might be just relaxing for a few minutes more before you drift
off . . . and that's all fine. . . . At home you'll be in your bed all
ready for sleep. But here you can choose how you wish to sit,
and listen, or even doze off a bit.*

I also suggest that some kids might listen to the recording more
than once as they go to sleep. Anxious kids, in particular, worry
that they won't be asleep by the time the recording ends. They
stay focused on their performance. Will they do it right? Will it
work? It's helpful to diffuse that from the start. Ultimately, the
goal is to fall asleep without the recording, but most will use it for
several weeks at least.

Induction

The focus of this session is creating an experience of physical variability (relaxation in this case) as well as loosening up rigid expectations
and beliefs about sleep. Thus the induction can simply set the stage
and invite the child to begin the process of settling in and shifting.

Some examples:

So here you are . . . cozy in your bed. . . . Move around and find a place that feels comfy . . . for now. . . . You will probably move around some more as you settle in . . . under the covers . . . and your eyes might be open or closed . . . and you can even take a nice deep, easy breath . . . as you start to slow down a bit. . . .

As you get cozy . . . find your comfy spot . . . you can close your eyes. . . . Your busy brain has learned so much today. . . . Now it gets to listen . . . drift along . . . and I'm going to tell you a story about a girl like you. . . .

Get comfortable in your bed . . . with your pillow and your blankets and your toy tiger you showed me . . . and together we can count from 10 to 1. . . . You can hear the numbers and even say them in your mind if you like . . . and with every number . . . your body gets a bit looser . . . slows down like the numbers I'm saying. . . .

As you listen to the sound of my voice . . . you can just adjust yourself as you like . . . starting to settle in. . . . Your body might move a bit . . . roll around . . . eyes open or closed or back and forth. . . . Some kids find a spot to stare at on the ceiling or the wall . . . or notice their eyelids getting heavy right away. . . . No right way . . . just a way. . . .

Building a Response Set

The goal here is to build responsiveness toward a flexible, natural shift or transition, both physically and cognitively, as needed. This is ultimately about moving more freely from being awake to being asleep, so start with a few truisms or generalizations about shifts that happen naturally and the variety of ways things transition from one state to another. In other words, there are many ways to get from here to there.

> *So you can get comfortable . . . little by little . . . or even all at once . . . just listening to me. . . . There are so many ways to do that. . . . You can listen with your eyes open or closed . . . or with your left ear or your right ear or both ears. . . . Think of all the different ways we do things!*
>
> *In the morning you might get dressed before you brush your teeth . . . or you might eat breakfast and then get dressed . . . and you can get dressed different ways on different days . . . as long as you leave the house with your clothes on. . . .*
>
> *And there are so many ways to make an ice cream sundae, or build a castle, or travel from here to California. . . .*
>
> *Kids are so different from each other in so many ways. . . . Some like running more than reading . . . or numbers more than letters . . . and some kids like cats better than dogs. . . . Kids learn in different ways, too. . . . Some kids learn to ride their two wheeler on the first try . . . but most have lots of stops and starts . . . and some things we learn to do without having to do much at all . . . like learning to eat a popsicle . . . or how to laugh. . . .*

The "I don't know" set described in Chapter 5 works well with the rigid child who, like Edward, is overmonitoring and watching the clock. Here we suggest that he can let go of that demand for now (and let's get rid of that clock):

> *I don't know if anyone knows how many ways there are to get comfortable . . . or how many little adjustments we make . . . or how many thoughts drift by . . . or when we stop noticing the sounds around us. . . . I don't know how we would even keep track of such things. . . .*

Interventions and Suggestions

The suggestions continue to build upon the themes of variability and flexibility as your words move more specifically toward relaxation and sleep. It's a process that waxes and wanes, so the tone is permissive and inclusive:

And as you relax your body . . . you can wonder . . . . if you'll feel most comfortable in your feet while your hands stay busy a bit longer . . . until they feel heavy too . . . or will your breathing slow down . . . or will your heartbeat get a bit slower? Tonight might be one way . . . and tomorrow a different way. . . .

I had a dog when I was a girl . . . and sometimes when she was getting ready to settle into her bed . . . she would walk in a circle one way . . . and other times she would walk in a circle the other way. . . . Sometimes twice around . . . sometimes once . . . and then she'd settle in . . . and let out a nice sigh. . . . She wasn't thinking about much . . . maybe her favorite place to dig in the dirt . . . or her favorite squirrel to chase . . . or her favorite sunny spot on the lawn . . . or the best crumb she found under the table after dinner. . . .

You can find your many ways too . . . sometimes moving around a bit . . . and other times feeling so heavy and tired in your muscles. . . . Sometimes imagining your favorite place to go . . . in your imagination . . . just noticing how your body sinks into the bed . . . that easy feeling of drifting around or sinking in. . . .

There's an old story about a boy and the sunset . . . and every night he watched the sun go down . . . and even though his teachers and his parents and the science books all told him there was only one sun . . . he couldn't believe it . . . because every night when the sun set . . . the colors were different . . .

and the clouds were different . . . and the sounds were differ-
ent. The summer sun was there so much longer . . . but the
winter sun left early in the silence. It's the same sun, but the
sun does it differently every night . . . always setting and always
rising . . . but painting a different sky each night . . . and a dif-
ferent dawn each morning. . . .

Michael Yapko uses these words to suggest that "in-between" place of transition: "And it's interesting . . . that as you drift off . . . you first find yourself . . . in this . . . in-between place . . . of not yet being asleep . . . and yet . . . not really awake either" (2006, p. 153). The normalizing of this transition between awake and asleep is often helpful. Many children have told me that this transition feels weird or scary, and they will force themselves awake when they notice it happening, or work hard to prevent it altogether. One child told me, "I just don't know how that works! How do I go from hearing to not hearing? I'm awake and then I'm asleep. It's scary that my body does that!" We came up with soothing and natural images to replace the scary thoughts, images of kittens and puppies falling asleep, and a calf dozing off in a summer field.

Children who have trouble initiating sleep at bedtime predictably have the same problem if they wake during the night (Meltzer, 2010). The skill of self-soothing and transitioning from waking to sleeping just isn't developed, or was developed and now has been disrupted. Every sleep session I do includes suggestions about returning to sleep during the night, emphasizing this normal and even predictable aspect of sleep.

And it's good to know . . . that your body makes adjustments
during the night . . . that you might turn over . . . or kick off your
blankets . . . even open your eyes and wake up a bit . . . and when
that happens . . . if you even notice . . . your body and sleepy

256

brain can make adjustments . . . just moving around while you settle back to sleep . . . finding your way back to sleep. . . . Once you know how to get somewhere . . . it's easier and easier to find it the next time. . . . You can count from 10 to 1 [or add the specific skills you've been working on] . . . while you drift back to sleep . . . again. . . .

Posthypnotic Suggestions

Because you want to end the session with a gentle, nonarousing good night that focuses on the present moment, weave the posthypnotic suggestions into the session, rather than as a more distinct ending to the session as described previously. Suggest future success and ongoing learning:

You are learning to be more flexible . . . letting your body and mind do what it does . . . here in this moment . . . and at the end of the day . . . night after night . . . sleep after sleep . . . morning after morning. . . . I wonder how you'll get more and more comfortable with getting comfortable . . . about sleeping . . . falling asleep and staying asleep . . . going back to sleep . . . knowing you can let it happen . . . in its own way. . . .

This first frame highlights the variability of experience in falling asleep, helping anxious kids such as Edward step out of rigid expectations and rituals toward the fluidity of sleep (and life in general). We want to introduce and normalize the concept of shifting and adjusting, so kids can learn to manage sleep without such pressure. We're not diminishing the importance of good sleep, but suggesting that healthy sleep, like a healthy diet or a healthy marriage, is more about flexibility than perfection. As Leora Kuttner (2009) observed, sometimes reliance on a sequence becomes a dysfunctional trap that impedes success and promotes rigidity.

But wait, you're thinking. Aren't routine and sameness and predictability important parts of sleep hygiene? What about families that are so loose or chaotic at bedtime that no one's getting good sleep either? Don't kids—including anxious kids like Edward—have thoughts, bodies, fears, and physical symptoms that need some structure and boundaries? Absolutely. And just as your healthy diet and healthy relationships combine reasonable flexibility with reasonable boundaries, the best sleep interventions require the blending of flexibility and boundaries. It is your job as the clinician to deliver the right ratio of each, depending on the child. The next frame focuses on parts, the frame I find most consistently helpful to families with sleep issues.

THE VALUE OF PARTS

Many of the interventions that focus on parts in the previous chapters certainly come in handy at bedtime. An anxious child can externalize her worry at bedtime in the very same way she does it at school. A depressed teen who is learning to disconnect from his globally negative thinking will certainly want to use that skill when he's trying to sleep. A child in pain, as she falls asleep or wakes during the night, benefits from shifting her focus or compartmentalizing her discomfort.

But nighttime, alas, seems to hold its own power, and the problems of the day are often magnified as kids and adults alike find themselves in the dark and the quiet. For a variety of reasons, we appear and feel less equipped to handle the fears, the problems, and the pain. Nighttime is when kids tend to go global, so in this next section I focus on several sleep-related issues that benefit from a hypnotically delivered parts perspective.

Sequencing and the Bedtime Routine

When children resist going to bed or falling asleep, the first point of intervention is the bedtime routine. Is it chaotic? Inconsistent? Has the child successfully learned how to stall with requests for more snacks, stories, screen time? Many parents also report the yo-yo problem: they put their child to bed, only to have her repeatedly get up, ask for something, or call for help. You may determine that the problem is a lack of routine or an inability for the child to fall asleep because, quite simply, no one has ever taught her how to consistently do it on her own. I find it helpful to ask the parents, "Do you think your child knows how to put herself to sleep at night? Has she ever been able to go from waking to sleeping at bedtime in her bed on her own?"

If together you determine that this skill has never been developed (for example, the child has always gone to sleep with an adult in the room, or routinely falls asleep somewhere other than her own bed and is moved), a sequencing intervention is a great place to start. Other factors may be contributing to the inability to initiate sleep, such as anxiety or fears, but let's focus here on the development—and hypnotic support—of the skill that teaches a child to move sequentially from one step to the next. In contrast to the focus on variability above, here we emphasize the benefit of linking one step to another step, in a predictable and ordered way for children with no self-directed routine. We'll deal with other impediments (e.g., fears, worries) in the next section.

The child who benefits from this frame, unlike Edward, isn't overly committed to a routine that isn't working. He isn't trying over and over as his frustration grows. This child doesn't even get started. While Edward is in bed, wondering why he can't fall asleep, this child won't go to bed alone in the first place and probably rarely has, except in circumstances of complete exhaustion.

Induction

An induction that seeds or models the upcoming focus on a sequence is best. Use the simple countdown described above, or any of the other inductions I've described in connection to the sequencing interventions. A progressive relaxation induction is an obvious choice because it focuses on relaxation and can be replicated easily and independently.

It's helpful ahead of time to ask the child what she does as she gets into bed (if she does) or what she can imagine doing when she's handling her own bedtime routine. Will she arrange her stuffed animals a certain way? Turn on the night-light? Put the cover over her hamster cage? Read a few chapters in her book? Turn off her phone (and all other electronics), turn the electronic clock around? These details will help you connect to her world and establish her routine.

Because the child is going to be listening to your session in bed, start by simply saying:

> *Now that you're in your bed . . . you can get comfortable
> . . . and maybe you've already pulled up the covers . . . and
> arranged your pillow. Maybe you've [preparation] . . . so you
> can close your eyes if you'd like . . . or find something to rest
> your eyes upon . . . like the glowing stars on your ceiling . . .
> and let out a nice easy breath . . . letting your body and brain
> know that it's time for a comfortable routine to begin. . . .*
>
> *You can start with the top of your head . . . and let each part
> of you get loose and relaxed [or you can squeeze your fists tight
> and let them relax and feel how warm they get]. . . . We've prac-
> ticed this before . . . so you can let your imagination do the easy
> work . . . and move, part by part . . . down through your body. . . .*

Building a Response Set Toward a Sequence or Routine

Offer truisms about the order of things, making sure to include examples of how things move from busy to quiet, or how we use routines to help us get from here to there, adjusting content and language to the age and interests of the child:

> *There's something nice about moving from one thing to another*
> *. . . knowing how something is going to go . . . how you move*
> *through a school day . . . or turning the pages of a favorite*
> *book . . . and already knowing what's on the next page . . .*
> *even the last page. . . . We all know how one thing reminds us*
> *of the next thing. . . . If I say A B C . . . your mind just goes on*
> *with the rest . . . and you don't have to think much. . . . The*
> *order is there . . . before you even finish thinking E. . . . Your*
> *brain already knows F G H I . . . all the way from A to zzzzzz*
> *[softly make the "z" sound and fade out]. . . .*

One 4-year-old boy I worked with was fascinated with construction. He knew the names of all the trucks and equipment, and loved playing with his collection of trucks. We talked rather casually about how the construction guys finish up the day at a construction site. The machines get turned off and the workers start packing up their gear. Step by step he described the process, ending with the quiet at night. The trucks need to rest before they work hard the next day, he told me, or sometimes they break down. I recorded the conversation and he listened to it as he fell asleep, often with a dump truck tucked under his pillow.

Interventions

Continue with language that suggests movement through a routine, becoming more specific about the helpfulness and pattern of a sleep routine that reminds our body and brains what comes next as we fall asleep.

> *And I wonder if, when you brush your teeth . . . you'll start*
> *to yawn . . . or when you smell your favorite blanket . . . your*

eyes close . . . getting ready in such an easy way . . . and little by little . . . parts of you start to rest. . . . Maybe your eyelids remind your chin or your jaw . . . and your neck reminds your backbone . . . and each breath in and out reminds your tummy . . . that it's time to relax . . . and all the parts say goodnight . . . while you just relax. . . . And just like you learned the words to your favorite song . . . you learn to get comfortable. . . . It happens over time. . . . It becomes easier and easier . . . like tying your shoes or blowing a bubble. . . . You get to figure it out . . . your own steps . . . a routine that slows things down . . . and lets you rest . . . and you can picture in your mind . . . whatever works for you. . . . Maybe you'll see yourself walking down a staircase . . . or floating from cloud to cloud . . . each cloud helping you feel sleepier. . . .

Or for the adolescent who needs a better sleep schedule:

You've learned the importance of going from one thing to another . . . more and more independently . . . sometimes without even thinking about it. . . . You get yourself from here to there . . . moving through the steps of a project . . . finding your way . . . your first job . . . training your puppy . . . so that it becomes automatic. . . . That's one of the benefits of being more mature. . . . You have so much more experience . . . experience you take from one place to help you somewhere else. . . . You become your own advisor . . . about the order of things . . . your order . . . so I don't have to tell you what to relax first . . . or what to shut off first. . . . You can discover . . . the order of your own falling asleep. . . . You decide if you'll relax your mind or your feet first . . . when you'll start the process of closing down for the night. You get to create your own relaxing routine . . . step by step . . . part by part . . . adapt-

ing and learning . . . knowing what's healthy . . . taking care of
yourself now. . . .

Posthypnotic Suggestions

As above, predict how the ability to fall asleep will continue to
improve, or wonder how all the different pieces and parts of what the
child is learning will work together.

So night after night . . . sleep after sleep . . . morning after
morning . . . as you sleep better and better . . . I wonder what
will start to come naturally . . . from all the things we've talked
about and all the stuff you've learned . . . about sleeping . . .
falling asleep and staying asleep . . . going back to sleep . . .
all the pieces . . . all the parts . . . relaxing together . . . drift-
ing off. . . .

COMPARTMENTS AND CONNECTIONS

As soon as you begin to create a consistent sleep routine with a
family, you are introducing the concept of compartments and differ-
entiation. You are in effect saying to the child, "Sleep time is separate from the rest of your day. . . . We are going to differentiate it by
wearing bedtime clothes, saying bedtime things, and creating distinct but flexible bedtime rituals and routines."

Sometimes, consistent behavioral management of a sleep routine
in the family is enough to resolve a child's sleep issues. Often, however, a cognitive, emotional, or physical problem is wrapped up in
the sleep disorder and needs attention. Whether the issue is developmentally normal (a child afraid of the dark or monsters, a teen
worrying before exams), or the result of another diagnosable problem (anxiety, depression, pain), using hypnosis to create compart-

ments—connections or disconnections—is essential. Let's look at how parts can be used to manage common sleep problems (often with the help of a bit of variability along the way).

Childhood Nighttime Fears

Nighttime fears are usually the domain of younger children, but can certainly show up in older children who see or experience something scary. When children are afraid to go to sleep, parents almost always jump in with reassurance: There is no such thing as ghosts. We lock our doors so robbers can't come in. I've looked in your closet and don't see any monsters.

The problem with this approach (other than the fact that it doesn't work) is that the parent is fighting imagination with reality and facts. (I heard one scared 6-year-old say to her dad, "You tell me there's no such things as monsters, but then you still look under my bed and in my closet! If they're not real, why do you look?") If facts alleviated fears, then everyone who drives a car would happily enjoy the safety of an airplane flight. Why would anyone who drives be afraid to fly, when we know statistically it's so much safer than driving?

In order to help a child deal with a scary imagination, we need to help her use her own imagination, as I often tell children, "for good rather than for evil." The goal is to help a child create distance from her own scary thoughts, whatever the content. Rather than being absorbed and overwhelmed, a bit of distance and a new perspective—along with a dose of humor, creativity, and independence—helps a child cope with the scary thoughts we all experience at times.

Holly, for example, was a 7-year-old afraid of the typical nighttime scaries. She refused to go to sleep alone and demanded the lights stay on all night. When she awoke during the night, she yelled until a parent came to her, terrified to get out of bed. More often than not, Mom or Dad stayed with her for the rest of the night.

When I met with Holly and her parents, they all agreed she had quite an imagination. Her nightly scary thoughts covered the gamut from ghosts to monsters to kidnappers to death. "I actually think Holly has a few imaginations," I told them. This captured her attention.

"I think you have different imaginations, like channels on a television or theaters at the movies. They're like compartments in your brain. You're fine during the day, right? So you must be able to imagine fun things and interesting things. You go into your helpful or fun imagination, like walking into the theater that's showing the movie you want to see with your friends. But at night, you step into your other imagination . . . where you imagine scary things . . . and you stay there! And watch the scary movie . . . or keep the television on the scary channel . . . and I think we should help you use your fun imagination at night, so the scary imagination can't be so powerful and bossy. . . ."

Holly—with her great imaginations—was able to absorb herself in ideas for using her fun imagination to quiet down her scary imagination. She decided that there was a boss of each imagination. The fun compartment was managed by her favorite movie princess. The scary compartment was run by a whiny, grumpy porcupine who didn't know how to make friends. We made a recording, telling the story of the two imaginations and their bosses. We discovered that the two bosses knew each other, and Holly decided they should become friends. She then decided the porcupine probably needed to go on a trip to learn how to be friendlier.

Armed with a new perspective on her scary thoughts, Holly listened to the recording at home. I told the family to keep tabs (with creative conversations at dinner, for example) on the porcupine and the princess. It was Holly's job to make sure the porcupine didn't take over again, and her parents could help with the stories about the porcupine's travels at bedtime.

Holly did not go home and happily turn off her light that first night. Nor did the yelling disappear immediately. But Holly and her parents now had a way to contain the scary thoughts using the very strength that made Holly so frightened in the first place. Holly improved steadily over the next several months as we made multiple recordings about the management of her imaginations. The family consistently used the strategies and had fun along the way, which made a big difference in their success.

For homework, I suggested two perspective-shifting books for the family to read together about nighttime scaries:

- *The Owl Who Was Afraid of the Dark* (2005), by Jill Tomlinson and Paul Howard, tells the story of Plop the young owl, who learns to see darkness as less scary when he experiences it from others' points of view. Darkness, he discovers, is helpful and important to many creatures, including owls. This book models the benefit of stepping back and looking at things differently, and of course specifically addresses the common fear of the dark.
- *Wanda's Monster* (2002), by Eileen Spinelli and illustrated by Nancy Hayashi, introduces us to Wanda, who learns a whole new way to handle the monster in her closet, and also learns that worries come, but worries go, too. The tone is playful and funny and shows kids how to view the monster in the closet from a different (and entertaining) point of view.

The Busy Brain

Holly's bedtime worries and fears were developmentally typical of children her age, and not evidence at that time of any other disorder. But what can we do for insomnia in children and teens that is indicative of depressed or anxious thinking? As described in Chapter 7, a pattern of rumination, or being stuck in one's own negative thoughts and perceptions, is a hallmark of anxiety and depression, and is present in children and teens (see, e.g., Nolen-Hoeksema et al., 1992; Michl et al., 2013).

Ruminating and falling asleep don't mix. At bedtime, the anxious ruminator begins to think about the risks of tomorrow: "What if I didn't study enough for the test?" "What if my dad doesn't pick me up tomorrow?" "What if I do something stupid at school?" And he may also replay the possible mistakes made that day: "Did I sound stupid when I said that?" "Why did my friend give me that funny look?" "Maybe when I said that it made my mom mad. . . . Did she look mad?" The closely related ruminations of the depressed child focus on his negative experiences: "I had a terrible day. . . . No one even talked to me"; "I did terrible on that test"; "I'm so sad my dad left"—and predict more of the same: "I can't go to school tomorrow. . . . It's so awful"; "My life is a mess. . . . Nothing will get better"; "No one will play with me tomorrow at recess. . . ."

Therapeutically, the larger goal is to help this child develop better coping skills, like problem solving or handling uncertainty, or developing a more flexible view of his life and the world. But this is not work to be practiced at night when trying to fall asleep. The goal, as Michael Yapko states, is to focus the child on something that reduces arousal and takes the mind in "utterly benign directions" (2006, p. 149). Yapko also makes the important point that focusing solely on physical relaxation is not enough when dealing with a ruminator at bedtime. It has been my experience that a child who is completely physically relaxed (using a progressive relaxation exercise, for example) is still quite capable of generating disturbing, negative, or arousing thoughts, and sometimes physical relaxation and calming create a quiet stillness that then enhances worried thoughts. Calming down the body is necessary, but your interventions will be more successful when they teach a child how to address her unhelpful ways of thinking about sleep and bedtime.

Again, compartments come in handy. Just as Holly learned she had different imagination compartments, kids (and especially teens) can be introduced to the idea of thinking compartments. The message is this: There are different types of thinking, some more useful than others, and you need to use the right type of thinking for the job at hand. I most often use this approach with children over the age of 10, so the examples below are aimed accordingly.

Induction

As you invite the child to tune in and focus on your words, immediately begin to suggest a separation, a transition to another way of being, thinking, responding, just as you would with most inductions.

> *As you settle in, you can take a few moments to shift into this part of your day . . . and congratulate yourself for a day done . . . however you did it. . . . I don't know what you learned in school . . . how many words you read . . . or math problems you worked on . . . how many instructions you followed . . . even when you didn't much feel like it . . . how many chairs you sat in . . . or conversations you had . . . or heard . . . or overheard. . . .*
>
> *Now isn't the time to keep track. . . . Who could, really? . . . All the different moments in a day. . . . Why don't you pay attention instead to letting go of any tightness in your muscles . . . letting your jaw and face and shoulders and spine . . . sink into your mattress and your pillow. . . .*
>
> *I know you have a busy brain . . . so many thoughts . . . ideas . . . questions . . . and for now . . . as you let those muscles relax and loosen . . . and settle into this part of your day . . . your good night . . . just let that busy brain buzz around for a while. . . . Even when we're not thinking . . . we're thinking.*

. . . It's just a different kind of thinking . . . and that's what I'm going to talk about . . . and you can listen . . . for a bit . . . and then listen a little less . . . and a little less. . . . There's different kinds of thinking . . . and listening. . . .

Building a Response Set Toward Selective Attention

Sometimes we do have to pay attention . . . when the teacher is talking . . . or we're learning to ride a bike or drive a car . . . or working on homework . . . but sometimes we can just space out . . . disconnect . . . like when we're hearing music in the background . . . or just hanging out with a good friend . . . the times when there's background noise . . . and it's just noise . . . nothing we need to do right then . . . nothing we really need to pay attention to. . . .

Interventions and Suggestions

Continue to build on the themes of disconnecting from problem solving or analyzing at night, while making suggestions to allow thoughts and words to float on by. Remember, we're not suggesting that the child needs to empty his mind, or relax, or even that he go to sleep. Instead of saying, "What you're doing [ruminating, catastrophizing, what-ifing] isn't working, so let's fix it" (you'll get to that in your daylight therapy sessions), this sleep session simply says, "Let's explore an easier internal place to be. . . ." The tone is one of allowing (versus doing) and finding a place that is distinct from the ruminating (M.D. Yapko, 2006).

There's a place we can go . . . in our minds . . . where thoughts and words and images . . . roll by. . . . My friend used to call it the easier place . . . because nothing there needed to be solved . . . or answered . . . and there was enough going on to keep her busy . . . in that different kind of way . . . like a silly movie . . . or a funny video . . . or [fill in known interest]. This same friend told me about her visit to a big art museum . . . and I don't know if you've ever been to an art museum . . . but you usually see people studying the paintings . . . and looking at the details . . . and talking about the artists . . . in a serious way . . . analyzing the details. . . . Perhaps they're studying for a test or writing a paper on a particular artist . . . and that's great for them . . . but my friend wasn't there to study. . . . She just wanted to stroll and look and wander. . . . She found a room with paintings and sculptures and photographs that were simply fun to look at . . . no work . . . no demands . . . not in this room. . . . She lost track of time. . . . Her brain was busy wandering . . . in such an easy way. . . .

And you might know about your easier place. . . . Maybe there's somewhere you go . . . a place in your mind where . . . your body relaxes . . . and you feel your blankets . . . and your pillows . . . where you don't have to do anything . . . where your mind is over here and over there . . . or thinking of this or that . . . or not much at all. . . . You don't have to know. . . . That's the easy part. . . . You don't need to know where your thoughts are . . . or how you'll start listening less. . . . You can just flow along . . . or wander . . . through the easy places. . . .

Posthypnotic Suggestions

The posthypnotic suggestion simply reinforces the ongoing experience of moving into the state of mind that is separate from the cognitive patterns of anxiety and depression as one falls asleep:

And whenever you listen to this . . . or remember this in your own imagination . . . as you discover you really only need to kind of listen . . . you can be so comfortable without knowing

*... or needing to know . . . or needing to think of much at all
. . . right now. . . . And when my voice stops . . . you can continue going along . . . in your own easy way . . . and feel so
rested . . . in the morning . . . with energy to learn and grow.
. . .*

I have a game that I often give to kids and adults to help them
become casually distracted as they go to sleep. Some kids use it without listening to a recording at all, while others use it after the recording is over. This is how I explain it:

*Pick a topic that you know fairly well. Dog breeds? Harry Potter
characters? Desserts? Baseball words?*

*Then, starting with A, or any letter you like, find a word.
Let's use desserts.*

*A? Apple pie. . . . B? Banana cream pie. . . . C? Chocolate
cake. . . . D? Devil's food cake, and so on.*

*Move along. If you come to letter and get stuck, just skip
over it. No pressure! You can go back if you think of something
later, but you don't have to.*

*So start with A or how about M? Mincemeat pie. . . . N?
Hmmm. Can't think of one. . . . O? Oreo cookie ice cream. . . .
P? Peach cobbler. . . .*

Pain and Sleep

Chapter 8 thoroughly discusses how to hypnotically help a child
cope with pain, but I'll offer a few more specific ideas about handling
sleep and pain.

Assuming that adequate evaluations have been done and medical
issues are being addressed, the most helpful and obvious intervention at bedtime is dissociation or disconnection from the discomfort.

Children who are beginning the process of managing their pain with hypnosis may worry that if the pain goes away at night (or any-time), then it's not real. At the same time, they may worry about how they will handle their pain if it occurs during the night when adults are not readily available. It is therefore important in the early going to be very permissive and inclusive about the pain's presence or absence during sleep and how they can manage their relationship to it. Make suggestions that foster curiosity and provide possibilities about how pain and the brain interact during sleep. Leave options open, focusing on modification rather than elimination of symptoms (Patterson et al., 2010).

I routinely include suggestions about pain's connection to sleep at the end of a pain management session. The session in its entirety teaches disconnection from the symptom or promotes an affective shift in relationship to the pain. You can certainly do a separate session focusing only on sleep. The suggestions about bedtime are an extension of the general theme of what we connect to, and what we move away from.

> *And when you're ready to sleep . . . when you're done learning and working and playing . . . getting cozy for the night . . . there are some things that are nice to notice . . . the feeling of your bed and your pillows . . . the places in your body and mind that feel comfortable . . . the way you feel when you're wearing your favorite pj's . . . or reading a story or two. . . . I used to read a book called* Where Does the Butterfly Go When It Rains? *. . . You might like that book, too. . . . It talks about where creatures go to stay out of the rain . . . and when I remember that book . . . it just makes me wonder . . . where does a tummyache go when you sleep? . . . I'm not sure what the answer is. . . . Maybe you already know. . . . Our bodies and brains do things a bit differently when we sleep. . . . We breathe more slowly . . . and we move a lot less . . . like a butterfly in the rain hiding quietly . . . resting its wings. . . .*

Our eyes don't see much, of course . . . and our ears don't
hear the littler sounds. . . . We notice some things . . . and
we make adjustments . . . when we need to . . . maybe a
tummyache goes to sleep . . . or maybe it comes and goes.
. . . You can imagine if you like . . . what yours might do . . .
when you're sleeping so deeply. . . . Where do you think it
might go?

Another approach is to hold a pre-bedtime meeting with the three interested parties: the child, sleep, and the physical symptom. With younger children this can be done with drawings or other props, and acted out in your office and then later at home if desired. (If you record it, they can listen at bedtime.) Older children can "go inside" and have the meeting, checking in with you as required. This is a perfect time to use the language of parts to figure out how the pain will be handled.

Neil was 10 when he broke his arm badly and required multiple surgeries. As he prepared for another procedure, he and his parents wanted to help minimize disruption in his sleep, an understandable problem following the past surgeries.

We set up a meeting with Neil, Sleep, and his Arm. Neil decided he would speak for Sleep and himself, and I would be the Arm and also play myself.

LYNN: So, we are here at the meeting . . . a meeting of Neil, his Sleep, and his Arm . . . so that you, Neil, can set some rules . . . so everyone knows what's needed. . . . Welcome Neil, Sleep, and Neil's Arm to this meeting. Neil, can you start the meeting by telling us what you would like?

NEIL: I would like to go to sleep and not have my arm wake me up.

LYNN: I see. A reasonable request, no doubt. Sleep, do you have any thoughts about this?

SLEEP (Neil): I don't want Arm to get in the way either. I'm Sleep, so

I want to sleep.

ARM (Lynn): Well, sometimes I just have to let you know I'm hurt-
    ing. What's wrong with that?

LYNN: Absolutely, Arm! We understand. But you need your sleep,
    too. You've been through a lot! I have to guess you'd like
    to be left alone sometimes, right? Sleep can help you feel
    better.

ARM: Yes, yes. I could use a break. Sorry. Bad joke.

LYNN: Neil and Sleep, what can we do here? Any ideas? Can you help
    Arm?

NEIL: Arm, I want you to go to sleep, too.

LYNN: Neil, can you and Sleep help Arm go to sleep? What messages
    can you send to Arm at night? What can you do inside?

Neil continued to talk with Sleep about helping Arm. With some
guidance, we agreed Sleep could send some extra Sleep Potion to
Arm. The Sleep Potion could move through his whole body, but an
extra dose would help Arm stay asleep. Arm expressed thanks:

ARM (Lynn): I could use some sleep, you know. . . . I don't want to
    keep us up, believe me. If I wake up at all during the
    night, just give me a little extra dose. Send some more
    my way.

LYNN: Sounds like we're all on the same team. Sleep, are you clear
    about your job?

SLEEP (Neil): I got it. I help Arm.

We recorded a brief practice of Neil instructing Sleep to send the
Potion. Neil decided to imagine his Sleep Potion as purple, and he
imagined seeing the purple potion moving into his arm. "That way
I can see where the Potion went and if I sent enough," he said. The
posthypnotic suggestions at the end of the recording summarized
the important points with predictions for success and some uncon-

scious dosing as needed:

> *So, Neil, it sounds to me like you and Sleep and Arm are on the same team . . . that you are tired from your day . . . and that you are all looking forward to getting some deep, comfortable rest . . . and that your Arm, too, understands that the healing happens all night. . . . And Arm is tired, too . . . and is so happy to get some extra Sleep Potion . . . and when you put your head onto your pillow . . . your eyelids and your legs and your spine and your feet and your muscles . . . will feel ready for sleep in a very good way . . . as you move the colored purple sleep potions to where they need to go . . . where you want them to go . . . and you can send more through the night . . . maybe even without waking up . . . while you close your eyes and rest . . . and sleep . . . until morning. . . .*

BRINGING IT ALL TOGETHER: NIGHT TERRORS, NIGHTMARES, AND THE THREE NEW FRAMES

Night terrors and nightmares in children have their feet firmly in the two camps of childhood development. Like insomnia, an occasional bout should be expected and normalized, but a persistent pattern becomes a problem that needs attention. In this final section, I offer ideas to help with both the occasional issue and the more serious problem. Not surprisingly, I've come across several innovative ideas for helping children with night terrors and nightmares, innovations that embrace the three frames of variability, parts, and action.

Night terrors are relatively rare in children, and most grow out of them by adolescence. They usually occur within a few hours after the child falls asleep. The child often appears terrified, screaming, thrashing, or running, with eyes open but not connected to his surroundings. The child does not respond to others, and adults can't seem to interrupt the episode or fully wake the child. After 10 to 20 minutes, the child returns to sleep, often with no recollection of what happened in the morning. Infrequent night terrors are not harmful and are usually left untreated. Parents benefit from information about what's happening and how to offer comfort during a night terror (ensure safety, offer comfort, don't actively try to realert). If night terrors become so frequent that they interfere with proper sleep, further evaluation and treatment are sometimes needed, as night terrors may be the result of fever, obstructive sleep apnea, restless leg syndrome, or migraines. Night terrors are sometimes connected to behavioral and emotional factors, such as poor sleep routines and resulting sleep deprivation, stress, fear, anxiety, or conflict (Sleep Terrors, 2014; Night Terror, 2014).

Assuming that medical issues have been ruled out or addressed, minimizing night terrors then involves educating children about sleep cycles, establishing proper sleep routines, and (if necessary) addressing any underlying emotional and family issues. Your job is to determine the best approach, and hypnotically you have some options.

If the sleep terrors are not indicative of psychological issues, you may take the concrete approach described by Kohen and colleagues, who reframed the episodes as "accidental bad habits" in the brain amenable to "reprogramming" (1992, p. 235). Treatment combined imipramine (a tricyclic antidepressant) and hypnosis, with suggestions for relaxation and the positive connection between brain and body: "Let some more muscles relax, nice and easy, because it feels so good, and because when you do this you get better and better at having that computer we call the brain and your body work together" (p. 236).

Kramer used a similar approach, using two sessions of hypnosis to educate a 10-year-old boy about the variability of sleep cycles and how to use them to prevent night terrors: "Upon completion of the induction, he was given an explanation of the nature of sleep, stage by stage. The regularity and continual movement of the cycles of sleep were emphasized. He was also given direct suggestions for not dropping too quickly into an extremely deep stage of sleep" (1989, p. 284).

There is little information on the treatment of night terrors that appear correlated with emotional or psychological issues (such as anxiety, stress, trauma, or family conflict), other than the general recommendation for further psychotherapy to address the source of the issue.

Taboada (1975) described his work with a 10-year-old boy that began having nightly terror episodes after returning from summer camp. He told his mother of a frightening experience on a sailboat, where the boys capsized in winds and waves. Everyone was fine, and Taboada used hypnosis to help the boy "perceive and imagine the danger situation differently" (1975, p. 271), connecting to an image of himself as older and stronger and able to manage the situation easily. Interestingly, the boy later confessed that the incident had never happened, but that he was afraid during a windy sailing episode and imagined what might happen. Taboada saw the night terrors as a fear of death, and the reconstruction of the albeit imaginary event resolved his fear and the terrors.

Nightmares are a normal part of development, experienced by almost all children at some point. But like night terrors, they can be an indicator of more significant psychological problems such as anxiety or trauma, a distinction based mainly on frequency, intensity, and repetitiveness of content (Mindell & Barret, 2002; Smedje, Broman, & Hetta, 2001).

When it comes to helping with nightmares, hypnosis shines. Whether the nightmare is the presenting problem or one of several symptoms, using hypnosis to address it results in a sense of confidence and self-control that, as we know, bleeds out into other areas. If the nightmare is the metaphor for a child's struggle, then rewriting and reworking it with hypnosis becomes a metaphor for mastery.

Rather than being a passive participant in the bad dream, the child actively shifts his stance and changes his position.

Kingsbury (1993) described his use of hypnosis to change the outcome or the characters in repetitive nightmares, regardless of whether the nightmare's content was based in reality or not. His goal was to take the client past the usual point of awakening and offer an alternative ending to the dream, one that would result in a feeling of mastery. He also described common suggestions to change the dreamer from victim to observer, disconnecting from the nightmare by viewing it on a television screen, adding commercial interruptions, adjusting the volume, or hitting a mute button.

McNeilly (2007) similarly described his approach to changing the content of a repetitive nightmare when helping a girl with a dream about sharks. He suggested posing a simple but solution-oriented question to himself and the child: What's missing? How can this child connect to her positive experiences and use them to alter the nightmare in some way? The girl, a Harry Potter fan, used magic to protect herself and frustrate the sharks.

Such techniques are helpful with repetitive nightmares, because you can hypnotically plan ahead and alter the familiar content. But what to do about nightmares that are not repetitive, or dreams whose content is barely remembered? Many children I treat report bad dreams (and a resultant fear about going to sleep), but the content is varied or generically scary. One approach, imagery rehearsal therapy (IRT), has been used with children (St-Onge, Mercier, & De Koninck, 2009) to "rewrite" a nightmare from the night before such that it is no longer frightening, and then rehearse the new version in their imaginations or verbally before bed the following night. Interestingly, kids did not report then actually having the amended dream, but did report more pleasant dreams and reduction in nightmares. St-Onge and colleagues concluded that it is not the incorporation of the suggestion that helped the children using IRT, but "the sense of control that appears to be the key mechanism operating in

IRT" (p. 95), namely the success with imagery control.

The term *hypnosis* is not used when describing IRT, but having a child create a different dream and then having her take action and practice this new story in her imagination meets my criteria for a hypnotic experience. The authors described the words they used: "It was suggested that there were thousands of ways of changing the nightmare, but that they had to personally choose one, try it, and if it did not work, change the nightmare in any other way" (St-Onge et al., 2009, p. 88).

I'm sure you must recognize this as a permissive directive to take action on a problem by flexibly creating a solution that would vary their dreams. Hypnotic, no doubt.

CASE EXAMPLE: MATTHEW WON'T GO TO SLEEP

Matthew's parents were having a tough time getting Matthew to bed at night. This was not surprising, as they admitted having difficulty getting Matthew to do much of anything on their terms. Five-year-old Matthew was funny and sweet and full of energy, but he also liked to be in charge—and could be explosive. His parents often felt like they were "containing not training" him, and they set the bar low. "We'll do anything just to get him to sleep," they told me. This meant bedtime was a circus of snacking, books, bed swapping, bathroom trips, and often yelling, in no particular order.

Matthew was an only child, and his parents told me they had never actually put Matthew in his bed, kissed him goodnight, and allowed him to fall asleep on his own. They had recently resorted to letting him stay on the couch with the television on, hoping he would fall asleep eventually. When he woke up during the night, he would call to his parents, who would bring him into their bed.

Matthew really had no idea how to put himself to sleep, nor did his parents know how to teach him. Based on Matthew's energetic personality and the chaotic disorder of bedtime and sleeping each night, Matthew needed a routine that would help him slow down and shift toward sleep in a predictable way, and learn the skills of falling asleep independently, both at bedtime and during the night.

I worked first with Matthew's parents on creating a consistent bedtime routine. We worked on standard behavioral changes, including making a list of the three things Matthew needed to do before bed (jammies, teeth, bathroom), and giving him the power to decide the order. His parents agreed to put him into his bed, read a story, turn off the lights, and then leave the room. They would stay upstairs until he fell asleep to start, and if he got up during the night they resolved to bring him back to his bed, no matter what. They were to remain calm and consistent.

The four of us met together and went over the plan with Matthew. He was agreeable with me, but he was generally agreeable with adults other than his parents. The family returned a few weeks later. After some initial resistance and admirable consistency by the parents, Matthew was doing much better staying in his room, but it was taking him up to two hours to fall asleep. I asked Matthew if he would like to record a story with me on my computer that would help him fall asleep faster. He happily agreed, and we sent Mom and Dad to the waiting room.

By the way, I have a big bin of very cool knights, horses, and other animals in my waiting room, and Matthew loved looking at them and arranging them.

Here's what we did together, all recorded for Matthew to use at bedtime:

Matthew, you have a lot of fun energy, don't you? You like to run and play and grow . . . and at school you're learning so many new things! Can you tell me what you're learning? [Matthew talks about the book his class is reading on planets.] Planets? Wow, do you know the planets? [He recites them.] Very impressive! So you know that some planets are close to the sun and some are far away? They're all lined up in order in our solar system, right? [He nods.] You must have a powerful brain to remember so many things, and powerful brains need to work and learn, and they also need to rest after all the learning. Kids' brains and grown-ups' brains need rest, and they rest at night, while we sleep. Did you know that? [Nods.]

Can I show you how I learned to rest my brain and my body, so I could learn and grow when I was a kid like you? I have a story to tell you about it, too, a story about a boy like you. I'm recording this on my computer like I showed you, so you can listen to this story whenever you like . . . but especially at bedtime . . . when you're cozy in your bed. . . . Okay?

First, we're going to start with a little slowing down so you can hear the story, like when you hear a story at school in circle and you listen so quietly. I'll show you. Let's sit here together and imagine our bodies getting comfy and relaxed . . . your arms and your legs and your fingers and your toes . . . your eyelids and your cheeks . . . your knees and your elbows. . . . You can let your body slow down . . . while you think of whatever you'd like . . . as long as it's something that makes you smile inside . . . maybe all those planets . . . or a place that you like to go. . . . Maybe you've been there before . . . or maybe it's just in your imagination. . . . Your body can start to get a little quiet while you imagine . . . and listen. . . .

I heard a story about a boy. . . . He had a lot of energy like you. . . . Can I tell you the story while you let your body rest? This boy was named Moe. . . . He was in kindergarten, like you . . . but he lived in a kingdom a long time ago. . . . His father was a knight who worked for the king . . . and when Moe got bigger . . . he was going to be a knight, too. . . . There were many things he needed to learn first . . . so he paid attention when his father put on his armor . . . and saddled up his horse . . . and did important jobs for the king. . . . Moe had to learn *so much! He decided that he would go to school during the day and learn how to be a knight at night. . . . He decided he didn't need sleep. . . . He had so much energy! For two weeks he didn't go to sleep. . . . When his mother told him to get ready for bed . . . he refused! When his father told him to brush his teeth and put on his jammies . . . he said no! They didn't know what to do because Moe was very loud and stubborn. He would fall asleep sometimes . . . but not for long. He felt tired . . . but he didn't want to tell anyone.*

Finally after three weeks, Moe's brain was so tired he couldn't learn and listen. His parents were tired too . . . but Moe wouldn't listen . . . until one night, the king came for a visit. . . . Moe knew the king because the king's twins, the princes of the kingdom, were in Moe's class at school and played on the same soccer team, and he had dinner at the king's fancy palace a few times. It was at bedtime . . . but of course Moe was still up. . . . The king went with Moe up to his bedroom . . . and helped him get tucked into bed. . . . The king had a nice smile . . . but a serious smile. And the king said to Moe. . . .

"I know you want to be a knight like your father . . . and you have energy and brains . . . and you learn things . . . but you cannot be a knight until you learn one very important thing . . . to sleep in your bed . . . to rest your brain and your body . . . so you can grow. . . . Your father is a knight. . . . He must sleep, too . . . so he can follow my orders and protect the kingdom . . . and your mother is the only person in the kingdom who knows where all the jewels and gold are hidden. . . . I have given her that job . . . so she must rest her memory while she sleeps. . . . Your whole family must sleep and rest. . . . You all have important things to do. . . ."

Moe was very quiet while the king spoke . . . but then he wondered . . . and he said to the king . . . "I haven't fallen

asleep on my own for days and days and weeks and weeks.
. . . King, what if I can't do it? What if I don't know how?"

The king pulled the blankets up to Moe's chin and handed
him his stuffed monkey. . . . Moe could feel how tired he was
. . . his muscles and his eyes . . . his legs and arms and brain
. . . and the king said to Moe. . . .

"You don't have to do a thing. . . . Your body already
knows how to fall asleep. . . . Ever since you were a tiny baby
. . . you didn't even know how to talk . . . or walk . . . or eat
by yourself . . . but your body knew . . . and you would look at
the ceiling . . . or out the windows of the carriage . . . or watch
the leaves on the trees . . . and all the while . . . your arms
and your legs and your tummy and your ears . . . they all knew
what to do . . . little by little . . . drifting off . . . while you just
thought your thoughts, which were hardly even words . . . and
it still works that way . . . and while you listen to my voice . . .
your body can remember what to do. . . ."

This is based on Erickson's (1979) early learning set described in
Chapter 5.

Moe felt better. . . . He did know what to do! . . . He just had to let his
body slow down . . . and let his thoughts wander . . . and bit by bit . . .
part by part . . . he would find sleep . . . and if he woke up during the
night . . . he could think about being a knight . . . or anything else . . .
while his body got cozy again . . . and fell back to sleep. . . .

And you, Matthew, are like Moe . . . smart and growing
and learning. . . . You know the planets and the alphabet . . .
and you need to rest your body and your brain . . . just like
knights and even kings. . . . Moe fell fast asleep . . . and you
can too. . . . You both know how that happens now. . . . So
good night, Knight!

Matthew enjoyed listening to the story. I also gave Matthew's parents the assignment of finding pictures of Matthew asleep in funny places as a baby. (If no pictures are available, I have parents tell the stories and then illustrate the stories together.)

We made a few more recordings over the next two months, usually about Moe and his adventures becoming a knight. It was tiring work, so Moe kept getting better and better at sleeping well. Matthew's bedtime routine was almost entirely resolved after the first recording. I think he just wanted to come back and play with the knights in my office.

CHAPTER *10*

Parents as Allies

*H*aving read this far, you are well aware of my emphasis on the influence and value of parents, and the importance of a family-based approach. From building rapport and gathering information during the initial contact to the varying roles of parents when addressing a child's anxiety, depression, or pain, I hope I have conveyed the value of understanding and incorporating parents in your hypnotic encounters. Gail Gardner wrote of inviting parents to be allies when using and teaching hypnosis, describing hypnosis as "an extension of natural parenting behavior" (1974b, p. 47) that lessens the helplessness parents feel when a child is suffering and creates a positive cycle of hope and mastery between parents and children.

The question for me is not whether to include parents in the use of hypnosis, but how best to include them. How can we help parents improve their communication with their children by using hypnotic language, casually or more formally? How can hypnosis and self-hypnosis bolster a needed connection (or healthy disconnection) between parent and child? When and how can we use hypnosis with parents to help with issues that impact their parenting and their children? Although I have talked about each of these throughout the previous nine chapters, this chapter concretely bundles them and allows me to offer a few final observations.

THE HYPNOTIC PARENT: SEEING A CHILD THROUGH DIFFERENT EYES

When people find out that I do hypnosis, they often jokingly say, "So do you hypnotize your kids?" Every chance I get, I tell them. The more accurate answer is that I attempt to consciously use hypnotic language as a way to communicate with my children, sometimes because it's fun and sometimes because I want to teach them something. (When they were little, I just wanted them to go to sleep.)

Many years ago I created a workshop for parents of young children called Quickly Calmer: Parenting Through the Tough Times. The overwhelming majority of attendees were parents with children ranging from 2 to 5 years old. Their children (as to be expected) were exhausting and challenging them, and they wanted to do more than punish, and yell, and corral.

We talked a bit about behavior modification techniques, but mainly focused on the power of language. I wanted to show them how to communicate with their children in a way that was absorbing and suggestive, like the previously mentioned story of Maria Montessori entrancing her class to listen to the baby's breath. My goal was to help them slow down and speak deliberately, with a focus on what they wanted to teach their child. What do you want your child to do? What did you need her to learn? Follow directions? Stop a behavior? Try something new? Go to bed?

In the few hours we had together, I focused on storytelling, changing one's tone, and using suggestions that fostered curiosity and problem solving.

- I wonder what we can do to get through the grocery store smoothly.
- I'm so curious about what we'll see when we drive to school this morning.
- I think we can get your shoes on. . . . Do you? What should we do?
- After we read this story, I think your eyes and your legs and your brain will be ready to just sink into your bed. . . .

I talked about modeling emotional regulation and slowing down:

- I am so frustrated right now, so I'm going to take a few breaths and think for a minute.
- I don't know what to do about that mess you made. . . . I'm not happy about that . . . so I need to take a moment and think before I talk.

I showed them how to do the simple Heavy Hands exercise (see Chapter 5) and encouraged them to practice it regularly, and use it in the moment when they needed a pause or a reboot.

> *You're standing in the kitchen and you're on empty. Your child has just pushed your last button. Rest your hand on the counter, make that hand heavy, and focus on your next move, on what you want to say and do as a parent in these few moments.*

I implored them to practice this together with their children, and conveyed the power of teaching young children a skill that fosters self-control and autonomy.

At the end of the workshop, I suggested they look for chances to see their children through different eyes, a stance of flexibility and variability that might break them out of reactive patterns (yelling, punishing) and enjoy parenting more. I then invited them into an experience.

After a simple and brief induction (often focusing on creating heaviness in their hands because I had just taught that to them), I said something like this:

> *And as you sit here . . . out of your normal routine on Wednesday night . . . I'm guessing the break in routine has been welcome . . . based on the many times we've laughed . . . and how willingly I see each of you . . . closing your eyes . . . settling in . . . and how just being here shows us both . . . your willingness to learn . . . to absorb . . . something new. . . .*
>
> *Parenting requires different things at different times. . . . No two children are the same . . . and no child stays the same for very long . . . as it should be. . . . You don't deal with your 3-year-old like you dealt with your newborn. . . . There's a flexibility that helps us navigate . . . their constant movement. . . .*
>
> *And this flexibility . . . whether it comes naturally to some of you . . . or is new to some others . . . allows you to adjust and adapt . . . as a parent . . . to respond to your child . . . to teach . . . to love . . . to set boundaries when needed . . . and to be spontaneous when you can . . . and so I offer you this little moment . . . to plant some seeds for a time in the future . . . when you'll be standing there . . . parenting. . . . Imagine that now . . . your child in front of you . . . perhaps in the midst of a challenging moment . . . a messy moment . . . a stubborn moment . . . an exhausting moment. . . . And you can take a few easy breaths . . . take your time . . . slow down for just an instant . . . and see your child looking back at you . . . waiting for your response. . . . Let your muscles and your breath and your thoughts ease up. . . . How will your words sound . . . even if you don't know exactly what you'll say? . . . What will your face say . . . in that snapshot . . . of waiting? . . . What happens*

*next? . . . Take your time . . . in the next few seconds . . . and see
your child through those calm eyes. . . .*

*I'll be quiet for a minute . . . and allow you to notice what
it feels like . . . to speak to your child . . . to think and imagine . . . how this can be for the both of you . . . to respond differently . . . the simple advice to think . . . and breathe . . .
and look . . . before you speak. . . . There's no rush here . . .
so enjoy the quiet for a minute. . . . [Silence for about one
minute.]*

*And wouldn't it be funny . . . before we finish here . . . to
even look forward to the next moment of messiness? . . . The
moment when your child looks to you . . . and you respond in a
different way . . . using your words to tell a story . . . or change
a pattern . . . to offer something in a way you both can use. . . .
I wonder when that will be. . . .*

*So when you're ready . . . you can end this brief experi-
ence . . . but take with you a different perspective . . . a perspective . . . a few ideas . . . a phrase or two . . . a heavy hand
and a lighter step . . . toward your child. . . . Take a breath or
two and open your eyes when you're ready. . . .*

In my experience, when parents embrace the use of hypnotic
language (and this means suggestive, imaginative, and positive language), parenting shifts from punishing and controlling to disciplin-
ing (teaching) and engaging. I urge parents to imagine talking to
children in a way that gets a child to step closer and listen. Hypnosis is a great therapeutic tool. When the parents learn how to use the
principles of engaging communication, they become better parents.

As I've described throughout this book, role-playing, personify-
ing parts, reading books together, and shifting the narrative with stories and metaphors are all approaches to model and teach to families.
One of my favorite homework assignments to illustrate the value of
hypnotic language is to have parents watch *Mary Poppins* and *To Kill*

a Mockingbird. If you haven't seen either film recently, I suggest you watch them, too.

PARENTS AND CLINICAL HYPNOSIS:
TO INCLUDE OR NOT?

Opinions about when and how to include parents in the use of pediatric hypnosis vary based on the presenting problem and treatment setting, but the general consensus promotes the reasonable stance that overinvolvement by parents negatively impacts success (Kohen et al., 1984; Kohen & Olness, 2011; Sugarman & Wester, 2013) while a supportive, collaborative approach that supports a child's efforts is often helpful. Linden (2011) wisely suggested that we consider the developmental age of the child, the reason for the hypnosis, and the psychological health of the family. Is there, as she described, a negative trance state, "an automatic pattern of communicating that keeps the dysfunctional behavior established"? (p. 72). If so, how can we use hypnosis with parents and children to offer new patterns?

The decision to include parents (and in what way), for me, relies broadly on a now-familiar frame: the role of connection and disconnection. Will the child's healing benefit from a fostering of connection, or more disconnection? Is the goal to create more autonomy and confidence in the child? How will the inclusion of parents support or sabotage this goal?

Let me offer some brief guidelines here, many of which will jog your memory based on my past examples more than offer new insights.

With younger children, parents staying or leaving is a clinical judgment call, but I often allow parents to stay for a brief demonstration unless there are clear reasons to dismiss them. (These include a parent who is intrusive, emotionally labile, or negative about the treatment.) A short induction followed by a simple suggestion and reorientation can do wonders to dispel myths and build rapport. If the hypnotic intervention is a seamless part of the session and the parent is not present, then stopping, inviting a parent into the room, and providing explanations just isn't necessary. Often, I simply ask kids (again barring any strong clinical reasons for parents to leave), "Do you want Mom/Dad to stay or shall we have them leave now?"

With adolescents, parents generally wait outside. If a parent has concerns or is curious, a quick demonstration helps. Some teens are happy to have their parents listen to the recorded session later "just to see what it was like," while for others, privacy is an important developmental and therapeutic stance.

The treatment issues being addressed also influence the parents' role. In anxious families, for example, creating autonomy and mastery is the name of the game. From the start, I want to promote the importance of the child being in charge of the tyrant called worry, and interrupt the common parental patterns of accommodation and external reassurance. I frame hypnosis as a tool to support courage and movement away from certainty and comfort (often provided by the parents). Therefore I keep parents at a bit of a distance. Optimally, this means the child practices or listens on her own, but for younger children, parents can cue or role-play the use of the techniques if needed. "That sounds like your worry bossing you around, so you can go inside and have a talk with that worry part. Using your imagination is your job." Because changing the catastrophic language, the overprotection, and modeling of anxious behavior in parents is such an important aspect of anxiety treatment, separate sessions with anxious parents are very valuable. I discuss how to conduct separate hypnosis sessions with parents for this and other issues in the next section.

The guidelines are similar for depression. Parents are in the room based on the age of the child, the nature of the session, and the parents' ability to support a more positive frame. For the most part, I want children to have an experience that promotes their ability to move forward and take action, and sometimes separating them from a parent's visible concern or own depressed affect is vital.

Children struggling because of family conflict or loss also benefit from some level of separation to help them see the possibility that their emotional pain will not always be so overwhelming. This can be hard to achieve with a parent present, as I discovered with a 10-year-old girl dealing with her parents' divorce and limited contact with her father. She wanted Mom to stay in the room during our session, but as I began talking to her about how she could miss her father and eventually begin to enjoy her friends and life, too, she opened one eye to glance at Mom. My ability to convey a new frame (that her parents' conflict didn't define all of her) was hindered in that session by her concern for her mother. "What if Lynn says something that upsets Mom, or makes her worry more? What if Mom gets angry or sad? Is it okay with Mom that I feel happy? Mom gets mad when I talk about missing Dad. . . . She wants me to be mad at him, too!" This certainly highlighted the need to address boundaries; therefore the hypnosis (and the therapy in general) focused on experientially conveying that to both daughter and mother, starting with separate sessions.

Chapter 8 discusses the interaction between children, parents, and physical or medical symptoms. Parents can play an influential role: positively as coaches and supports in using hypnotic techniques, negatively as models of catastrophic and somatic patterns of coping. Generally, the relationship between parents, pain, and children becomes more complex with chronic pain. Multiple studies show that a parent's catastrophizing predicts greater pain-related disability, somatic symptoms, and depressive symptoms in teens (see Lynch-Jordan, Kashikar-Zuck, Szabova, & Goldschneider, 2013; Wilson, Moss, Palermo, & Fales, 2014). However, parents enlisted as helpers who can cue and guide their children as they prepare for surgery or other procedures create not only positive connection but a shared sense of purpose in an often frightening situation.

Are all parents capable of playing this role? Of course not. I remember one mother who had great difficulty with her daughter's upcoming surgery. My hope was that giving Mom instructions on modeling and cueing some relaxation prior to and after the surgery would interrupt her "worry chatter," but it was clear almost immediately that Mom was not able to disconnect from her own worry even in the presence of her daughter. The best solution was a recording that I made with the daughter and a pair of headphones to listen independently.

On the flip side, I have found that some nervous, even catastrophic parents can shift out of this pattern when I talk to them about the inevitability of their understandable worry and the benefits of a different approach. I say directly, "It would be strange if you weren't worried and scared. I want to show you how to disconnect from your own worry for a bit and channel your concern. By helping with some exercises, you can be loving and responsive in really positive ways. I want you to focus on coaching your child, which will help you all feel more capable of handling this."

HYPNOSIS WITH ADULTS TO ADDRESS PARENTING ISSUES

On a regular basis, parents express gratitude for being able to use the skills I'm teaching their children to their own benefit. Anxious parents learn by proxy to externalize their own anxiety and respond more flexibly. A father who struggled with sleep took the strategies I taught his son and applied them with success to his own "busy brain." And because I also work with adults, sometimes the benefits go in the other direction as well. A depressed and pessimistic woman I was treating learned how to offer alternative perspectives to her globally negative teenager, and a young mother with her own abusive childhood began to use hypnotic and positive language with her twin toddlers because, she told me, she recognized what it felt like when I talked to her in that way.

Obviously when you help an adult with her depression, anger, anxiety, or pain, you are helping her family. Whenever we work with adults, we hope that the benefits roll downhill. So before we leave the topic of hypnosis and parents, I wish to offer you some examples of interventions I use with my adult clients that are aimed at common parenting struggles, some that are universal issues and some that are hallmarks of the times we are living in.

Connecting and Disconnecting

Several years ago I was listening to a program on my car radio. The first versions of what we now call smartphones were taking the business world by storm, and a working mother of a 2-year-old was describing the moment she recognized its impact on her parenting. While sick in the bathroom with food poisoning, she confessed her toddler retrieved her device and brought it to her, sweetly holding it out and asking, "Feel better? Feel better?"

Looking around, I see more and more of what can only be described as distracted parenting:

- Children who are trying to tell Daddy that they have just dropped a mitten on the sidewalk, while Dad marches on, looking at his phone
- Minivans equipped with individual screens for each child in the back, so they not only don't have to talk to their parents, but they no longer need to interact with each other

I don't mean to sound like the grump, pining for the good old days, but the importance of connection in parenting seems rather timeless to me, not something to be considered a casualty of "progress."

Paradoxically, I have story after story of parents keeping track of their children's every move, texting constantly, monitoring homework assignments and grades online, and having cameras installed at home so parents can watch children on their phones wherever they are and whenever they want.

A hypnosis session that focuses on the parenting balance between healthy connection and autonomy is applicable to adults who are:

- Dealing with their own anxiety or struggle with rigidity and perfectionism
- Have a child dealing with anxiety
- Stepping into a more involved parenting role because of divorce or custody changes, adoption, or remarriage
- Handling a change or transition in the family, such as a move, new job, or a child starting high school or college

Use the session to illustrate the movement between stepping in and letting go, and how awareness of oneself and children is needed to develop this skill. The goal is to offer examples of how both connecting and disconnecting can be done in a healthy way, and to create flexibility where there may be rigidity, fear, or a lack of confidence and experience.

The induction can simply suggest a relaxing adjustment that previews the theme of connecting and disconnecting:

> *Go ahead and take a few breaths, noticing how an exhale or two can settle you into this experience . . . and how you might notice the way your arms are resting . . . or your position in the chair . . . and giving yourself a moment . . . or two . . . as you listen to the sound of my voice . . . to let go of any obvious tension in your body . . . and noticing how you can notice less and less of the outside world . . . so you can have this experience . . . my words . . . your thoughts . . . separate from your busy days and connected in a different way. . . .*

The response set builds on these ideas of connecting and disconnecting and the challenge of sorting through the options:

And there's so much to pay attention to . . . many small details and bigger concerns . . . calls that require our response immediately . . . and other requests that can wait . . . combined with things that sound important . . . feel essential . . . but really don't matter much in the long run. . . . It can sometimes seem that everyone wants a piece of you . . . while you just want to make sure nothing falls through the cracks . . . the mixed messages that tell us to take charge but preach the value of letting go . . . of being in the moment and planning for the future. . . .

The interventions and suggestions then move more specifically into parenting, suggesting the balance one can strive toward through experience. Provide examples of both positive and negative connections and disconnections, and the inevitability of mistakes and adjustments. Anxious, fearful parents need more emphasis on the importance of letting children learn their own lessons, tolerance of uncertainty, and the value of failing. Busy, stressed, or emotionally disconnected parents need concrete examples of what true connecting might look like.

And when it comes to parenting . . . the messages can be just as confusing. . . . We're responsible for their well-being. . . . We want them to be happy . . . and to succeed, too. . . . How much do we help and push? . . . And when do we back off? . . . Sometimes kids learn so slowly . . . and we want them to speed it up . . . to our pace . . . and other times they want to charge ahead . . . and we want to hold them back. . . . Is this when you let them learn the hard way . . . or when you step in to save the day? . . .

We connect and disconnect . . . over and over . . . stepping in and stepping back. . . . If you watch the toddlers at the playground . . . you'll see them coming in for a quick touch . . . a pat . . . an announcement . . . the shared smiles. . . . "Watch me, watch me." . . . Then running off again . . . to climb on their own . . . and compare that to the parent on the phone . . . sitting in the bleachers . . . or at the concert . . . there but not there . . . not able to cheer and hear . . . the voice mail coming in. . . .

It's not about doing it right in every moment . . . but catching the moments . . . when connection is needed . . . and those moments might be fun . . . or they might be painful. . . . When all the distractions are muted . . . and when your focus is clear to you both . . . and there are the moments, too . . . when it's best to disconnect . . . to let go . . . with equal focus . . . giving the message to your child . . . "You can do this." . . . We've all held on too tight at times . . . and we've all tuned out too soon . . . even in our most mindful moments. . . . We've overstepped . . . or underestimated. . . . There's no perfect balance. . . . It's about making adjustments . . . moving out of balance and then noticing and practicing how to find it again . . . a series of moments and adjustments. . . .

And even sitting here . . . you can allow yourself to imagine those moments. . . . Maybe they are easily recalled . . . a part of your experience . . . the ones where you allowed yourself the time to listen or watch . . . or maybe you can begin to create them . . . to imagine them and practice them . . . to begin the process of sorting through and quieting down enough to imagine . . . the holding tights and the letting go's . . . that add up to something. . . .

Check in here with an open invitation:

And in a moment I'm going to check in with you . . . and if there's anything you'd like to share or ask . . . you can let me know. . . . I'd be curious about what you're thinking about or experiencing. . . . You can talk to me while staying just as focused as you've been for the last several minutes. . . .

After listening and processing as needed, suggest a return to a focused state and offer posthypnotic suggestions to reinforce the message, utilizing the feedback from the client:

> *You've been able to take this experience and revisit [or imagine] moments of connection and disconnection . . . and based on our conversation . . . it's nice to hear how you [recap experience]. When you open your eyes in a moment . . . and later today . . . and over the next few weeks and months . . . you can be aware of how many more moments are ahead of you . . . how many opportunities to pause and listen . . . to step in or step away . . . and I can only imagine . . . and you can only imagine . . . how that will go . . . smoothly sometimes and trickier sometimes . . . finding the balance between you and your children . . . being there in many different ways . . . as they change and you change . . . moment by moment. . . . So take some time now to begin to reorient yourself. . . . Take your time. . . . Connect fully again to this room and my voice . . . opening your eyes when you're ready. . . .*

Boundaries Between Then and Now

Closely allied to the issue of connecting and disconnecting is that of boundaries in parenting. This becomes my most pressing target when a parent is struggling with her own issues and needs an intervention that helps her differentiate between her own issues and her parenting. Sessions targeting the issue of boundaries are most often done with adults I am working with individually.

Remember Ellie from the start of Chapter 8, whose parents' ongoing conflict and emotional fragility were impacting her chemotherapy? If either of Ellie's parents were my client, I would have done a session focusing on behavior in the various compartments. To me, there were obvious compartments: parenting Ellie through her leukemia/chemo compartment, the marital conflict compartment, and maybe even a compartment for when Ellie was not in the hospital and was doing well, to introduce some fun and lightness into the family interactions.

Caroline was another parent who needed help with a boundary. Although she originally came for consultation about her daughter's anxiety, it was clear to us both after our first session that her own childhood greatly influenced how she parented all three of her children. Her daughter was hankering for some independence, but was not able to move past Caroline's catastrophic warnings, and consequently we agreed to focus on differentiating her own upbringing from her current role as a mother.

During Caroline's childhood, the world was a dangerous place and she couldn't count on her mother to protect her. Her goal, she said, was to make sure that her children always felt loved and secure, but this had led to extreme overprotection and fear. Our brief work together focused on separating her childhood from her children's and creating a new definition of mothering that allowed for love and independence. Using hypnosis, Caroline was able to put her childhood "over there" and her current family life "right here." Posthypnotic suggestions reinforced her ability—when she recognized that she was overstepping or catastrophizing—to see her childhood as a part of her past that was on the other side of a wall. The height of the wall was in her control, and she "built it up" when she needed to separate from her own childhood and give her children "a longer leash." She ultimately learned to accept a certain amount of risk in the name of healthy autonomy for her children.

Compartments and Conflict

The impact of parental conflict on children is well known. Often, however, despite the promises and intentions of almost all warring parents to keep their children out of their conflict, the reality is quite different. Compartmentalization is a frame that serves families well with parents that are enmeshed in battles with each other. Whether parents are together, divorcing, or already divorced, this frame helps parents recognize the need to protect children from adult issues and conflicts. Prevention is ideal, but more than likely you will introduce the frame as a way to interrupt a pattern of putting the children in the middle of parental conflict. The use of hypnosis has great potential here as an indirect approach that bolsters the direct instructions most parents have already received from multiple sources. A less confrontational, less directive approach may allow warring parents to shift their frame from combat with the other parent to compassion for their child.

Bob and Meredith, for example, had been legally separated for several months, but were both still living in the family house as they fought their way through a contentious divorce. They sought help for their son James, who was angry and disrespectful to both of them, with increasing episodes of raging and destructive behavior at home. Police had been called and inpatient treatment was being considered. The family doctor had already prescribed antidepressants for this "uncontrollable" 11-year-old boy, even though neither his teachers nor his coaches had seen any evidence of this behavior.

I agreed to meet with the two of them to determine if I could help James. The hostility in their relationship was clear from the few e-mails we exchanged while setting up the appointment, but even so, the unspoken vitriol between them as they entered my office was unsettling. I could only imagine what it was like for their son to be in that house with them both.

After talking to them together for a few minutes, I'd seen and heard and felt enough.

I asked to speak to each of them separately. Knowing they had already attended mandated classes on parenting and divorce and that the doctor and lawyers had already addressed the impact of their conflict on James, another lecture would likely do nothing. How could I get the message across, one that seemed so obvious (probably even to them) but that had not produced any changes in behavior? The father was successful in sales and the mother worked at a nursing home, so, using their professional strengths, I said something like this to each of them individually:

I know you've been going through a lot. . . . I'm guessing you're probably exhausted from this situation. . . . You've gotten a lot of opinions from many people . . . but I'd like you to listen for a bit . . . take a break for a few minutes. . . . I can see how tense this is. . . . Maybe you haven't taken a break from it in awhile . . . so I'm asking you to hear this perhaps in a different way. . . . Just breathe for a moment. . . . Slow down just for a few minutes. . . . I know you're very concerned about James . . . and rightfully so . . . as you sit here now and think about what it must be like for him . . . to watch his parents battle . . . what he's heard and what he's seen . . . being in the middle. . . . I've been a therapist for over 20 years . . . and being between the two of you has been tricky for me . . . but as an adult I can step into my therapist role . . . be here in this office and send [your spouse] into the waiting room. . . . Those kind of compartments come in handy. . . .

It's interesting how often people tell me that they feel something all the time . . . or that they can't control their reactions to things. . . . Maybe James has told you this after he's exploded or misbehaved . . . that he can't help it . . . and maybe you've told yourself that you can't help but be angry toward [spouse] . . . but just as I have this office and this waiting room and my role as a therapist . . . I know you have a job . . . where you successfully step away from the conflict and emotions of your divorce . . . where you treat people differently . . . respond differently . . . because sharing your anger about your divorce has no place in your workplace. . . . It

would damage your career and the people around you. . . .
Your feelings aren't your chief concern . . . or the concern of
your [clients/patients] . . . and it's a valuable skill to have . . .
the ability to step outside of your anger . . . your divorce . . .
and step into a different compartment . . . a different role . . .
when you have to . . . when you need to. . . .

Most people have many roles . . . as employee or boss
. . . son or daughter . . . sibling . . . partner . . . friend . . .
and parent . . . and being able to separate your roles . . . to
step away from one and into another . . . this has to happen
now with James. . . . Step into your parent compartment . . .
where you focus on your son . . . when you are in the house
. . . his home . . . and see things through his eyes . . . just as
you do with your [clients/patients] . . . because when he is in
the divorce compartment with you . . . of course he's angry and
out of control. . . . That's what surrounds him in that compart-
ment. . . . Imagine how that surrounds him . . . swirls around
him . . . and imagine how he feels and behaves when he's sep-
arate from that . . . playing with his friends . . . or continuing to
enjoy school. . . . He doesn't need to be in that compartment.
. . . He shouldn't have to be in there with you. . . . I don't know
how long you and [spouse] will choose to share this compart-
ment . . . but I am asking you respectfully . . . in a way James
can't because he's a child . . . to leave him out of this. . . .

I was acutely aware of being hypnotic during these conversations.
I slowed my voice, framed this conversation as a break from their
globally contentious patterns, and worked to offer each of them
images of compartments that were positive and accessible. Both
parents loved James and were able to appreciate the importance of
respecting his "son" and "boy" compartments, distinct from their
"battle" compartment.

I agreed to work with James. I taught him the same language

of compartments, helping him see that he could step into his friend compartment or school compartment (as he already was doing successfully at times), and coaching him to directly tell his parents that he wanted no part of their battle compartment. His parents learned (slowly) that his rage appeared when they tried to pull him into that compartment; and like a cat being dragged into a swimming pool, he fought back. Not surprisingly, when the parents moved into separate houses, things became easier. They remain angry at each other, but have done somewhat better keeping James and other family members out of their bitter relationship compartment.

Hypnosis Bolsters Behavioral Plans

In Chapter 5 I described my use of brief 3–5-minute recordings, particularly with younger children, that serve as reminders of what we did in the session. After we come up with a plan to handle a trip to the dentist or get on the school bus during the session, the recording is there to reinforce how to battle the worry bug and to activate those tools in the moment.

The same technique can be used when helping parents stick with a behavioral plan. I often meet with parents who need better nighttime or morning routines. Perhaps the parent is a procrastinator who invariably ends up yelling to get everyone out the door on time, or has a hard time tolerating whining and crying and consequently gives up on implementing a consistent bedtime. The plan itself is usually straightforward and seemingly easy to implement as we discuss it sitting in my office, but support and some mental rehearsal are needed at home, when reality hits and old patterns tempt.

At the end of the planning session, I propose to the parents that we take a few moments to review and mentally rehearse what we've come up with. I record this short review that is concrete in its instructions (sequencing), connects them to the positive experience in the office of creating a viable plan, and suggests positive expectations for consistency and success. Parents can listen to it when they need to—before or during their challenging parenting moments. And there will be challenging moments, especially during the initiation of new routines.

The simple format looks like this:

- Instruction to focus internally for a moment and reconnect to the plan that you've created . . . through a few simple breaths, a countdown, or another simple cue.
- Reminder of the importance of the plan and why the parent is working to make the change: "And as you take those breaths, you can be fully aware of how important it is to you and your children that the mornings go smoother, and how you'll feel when you say goodbye feeling positive and competent . . . and the value of role modeling [new routine]. . . .
- Take a simple walk through the steps of the plan.
- Posthypnotic suggestions that emphasize the positive results of following through and movement from conscious practice to more automatic patterns in the parents and children: "Take a moment now to move forward in time a bit and see for yourself what a smooth and organized morning will be like . . . how your voice will stay calm . . . how you yourself will stay on track . . . moving from one step to the next . . . and remind yourself that like your other successes . . . this process becomes more automatic with time and consistency . . . that you and your children can find a rhythm . . . that will build on itself . . . momentum in that positive direction . . . that's familiar to you from [fill in other successes]. . . ."

CREATING A HEALTHIER START

I have focused in this chapter on working with parents in conjunction with their children, and also on how to target interventions with adult clients that ultimately will help the children who depend on them. In an ideal world, whenever we enhance parents' well-being and connection to their children from the start, we are hopefully preventing many issues from developing in the first place.

One of my great joys is using hypnosis with pregnancy and childbirth. My own experience using hypnosis during the births of my two sons and my subsequent work with many, many pregnant women and their partners has shown me the value of hypnosis in creating positive expectancy, promoting a connection to the baby and the birth process, helping with healing, and supporting more confident nursing.

Luckily, there are multiple resources for clinicians and parents who want to use hypnosis to create the positive frames that should welcome all babies into the world. Hypnosis for childbirth classes are offered in many hospitals, and several books and CD programs are available for use at home. My colleague, psychotherapist Helen Adrienne (2010), author of *On Fertile Ground: Healing Infertility* teaches hypnosis and mind-body approaches to help couples navigate the emotional roller coaster of infertility (her website is Mind-Body-Unity, www.mind-body-unity.com). Another colleague, Dr. Sara Rosenquist (2010), wrote a terrific book called *After the Stork* that offers concrete strategies for new parents. It is preventative and positive, while normalizing the reality of this huge life adjustment. (Hint: it's not all about the hormones, as evidenced by the number of men also struggling with postpartum depression.)

Hypnosis stands in contrast to the culture of fear and worry that so many expectant and new parents experience. I have had plenty to say on the patterns of children's depression, anxiety, and pain and the frames we can use to interrupt them. I urge you to explore how these very frames can also help women and their families positively navigate pregnancy, childbirth, and the remarkable shifts that come with parenthood. Helping new parents develop or strengthen their resources from the very start is, in my opinion, one of the most valuable uses of the positive and active approach that hypnosis inspires.

Subsequently, these skills are carried into each new stage of development, with adjustments and tweaks here and there, but with the sustaining and overriding themes of teaching, moving forward, and discovering independence.

CHAPTER *11*

Spreading the Word, Hypnotically

*A*s I was writing this final chapter, a 12-year-old girl and her parents came to see me for the first time. The girl was almost completely recovered from a significant illness, but the symptoms had heightened her well-established anxiety about sickness and her body, and she had developed more and more somatic symptoms over the last few months. I asked her what she thought about our appointment together. Her mom quickly chimed in, "She was fine until I told her you do hypnotism. Now she thinks you can read her mind." Sigh. This led to an educational conversation about my use of hypnosis, a great opportunity to dispel myths and begin building rapport. But it confirmed what I already knew: the misconceptions regarding hypnosis are nearly as common now as they were 20 years ago when I began learning about hypnosis myself.

Hypnosis, as most of us are well aware, is routinely portrayed in movies and television as powerful, mysterious, or scary. In her

2006 article "Hypnosis in Film and Television," Deirdre Barrett listed 230 films that include hypnosis. The overwhelming majority portray the hypnotist as "larger than life and usually up to no good" (p. 26). Most of the hypnotists are controlling their subjects in the name of murder or other crimes, or for sexual purposes. The emphasis is almost exclusively on the power of the hypnotist to get his (or rarely her) needs met.

On the surface, I suppose a movie about a child using hypnosis to manage anxiety or deal with migraines is far less exciting than *Shallow Hal*'s depiction of Tony Robbins hypnotizing Jack Black's character Hal in an elevator, resulting in Hal's ability to see an obese woman as a beautiful, thin, blonde Gwyneth Paltrow. But as I watched *The King's Speech*, which in 2010 won four Academy Awards and was a popular and critical success, I noticed with delight the use of hypnotic language, indirect suggestion, rapport, and some strategic brilliance by speech therapist Lionel Logue as he helped King George VI overcome his debilitating stutter. (And let's not forget Mary Poppins.)

Because of its reputation and portrayals, *hypnosis* is not a neutral word. As I said in Chapter 2, the use of the term has the ability to create positive placebo and expectancies, as well as reactions of distrust or skepticism. It is a word that gets people's attention. But despite the negative portrayals and misconceptions, evidence and anecdote support my belief that when you talk to people who work with children about hypnotic techniques and language, many recognize elements of what they already do, and welcome more information and exposure to enhance their skills; clearly there is opportunity and demand for instruction and further dissemination of this valuable tool.

Almost thirty years ago, Gail Gardner (1976) surveyed child health care providers ranging from pediatricians to nurses to psychologists and discovered that attitudes about hypnosis with children were predominantly positive. But many were not fully aware of how hypnosis could be effectively used with children. And all groups of respondents (even those in the mental heath field) considered hypnosis more appropriate for medical problems than emotional, behavioral, or developmental problems. The limited view of hypnosis's versatility is also evidenced by the lack of literature on the use of hypnosis with childhood depression, and the frequent focus on symptom resolution (for example, with anxiety) rather than on broader skill building with children.

At the same time that Gardner was surveying her colleagues about pediatric hypnosis, Karen Olness (1977) reported on the results of multiple staff trainings at the Minneapolis Children's Health Center. She found that these trainings led to an increased awareness and an appreciation of the formal and informal benefits of hypnotic language and techniques. In 2003, Linda Thomson described the impact of providing accurate information about using hypnosis with children to 300 health care workers, 70% of them nurse practitioners. The presentation, according to responses from participants, led to increased enthusiasm for more training and use of hypnosis in clinical practice. Before the training, 29% stated they would suggest hypnosis to patients; after the presentation, 83% said they would. At a 3-month follow up, 56% reported they already had done so. Importantly, Thomson observed the recognition among many health care workers that much of what they were already doing in their practice was hypnotherapeutic.

So let's spread the word. Hypnosis is a valuable tool that creates transformative experiences, both in our offices and out in the world. It need not, and should not, be separate from anything we do in our treatment of children. The more we include other professionals in the use and delights of hypnotic communication and skill building, the more children will benefit from all that it offers. Yapko said it well in his article "The Spirit of Hypnosis: Doing Hypnosis Versus Being Hypnotic":

I would like us to quit putting obstacles in front of other professionals who want to learn and use hypnosis. Instead of increasing the hours for certification and consultation, thereby making it harder, and scaring people with stories of all the dangers of hypnosis, I think we should be making it easier for people to join, easier for people to see and enjoy the merits of employing hypnotic approaches. (2014, p. 243)

What gets in the way? The need to see hypnosis as distinctly separate from what we do with children. Iserson (2014), for example, looked at the use of hypnosis in emergency medicine. Despite long-term and successful reports on the benefits of hypnosis in emergency and medical settings, including its use with children, he concluded that acceptance and use "will require research into the most effective techniques, delineating in which acute care situations, where it is most effective, providing education and training in hypnotic techniques, and, eventually, its endorsement by major professional organizations and inclusion in required curriculums" (pp. 593–594).

The position I hold, and hope I've conveyed clearly in this book, is that you can and should develop your ability to consistently fold hypnotic techniques into your work with children. No hypnosis consent forms. No disclaimers. Get better at helping children by learning and practicing how to communicate in engaging, creative, compelling ways, and make hypnosis a part of that treatment. Pay attention to the power of suggestion, both negative and positive. Take the time to finesse and garner this power by learning and then amplifying your ability to move children toward mastery. I urge you to pursue your own professional development in hypnosis and use of these skills in the very same way you responsibly develop and engage in every aspect of your profession. Appendix A lists further training options for all levels. There's nothing like being surrounded by expert, enthusiastic teachers and fellow learners to boost both your skills and confidence.

The goal is to use hypnosis in the way that works for the child in front of you. Sometimes the ritual enhances the experience. It's why some religions build massive, beautiful churches and hold glorious ceremonies at specific times, and why many cultures have ways to send boys into manhood and girls into womanhood. Many human beings like to mark a shift in some memorable way that makes it more powerful, with absorption in stories, sequences, and connections that convey a message. Apparently, just saying "be nice to that other guy" or "time to grow up" or "the earth just made another one of its trips around the sun" just doesn't always deliver the message with the gentle jolt needed to get someone's attention or impact behavior.

And, paradoxically, sometimes it's not the ritual at all. It's not the bigness of the ceremony or the expected routine of closing one's eyes and counting from 10 to 1 that causes the shift. Instead it's a seed that's dropped, or a surprising, unexpected comment that jars a child's awareness, disconnects him from his normal patterns, and allows him to have a different experience, like when:

- You are quiet instead of loud to get the attention of a room full of children (like Maria Montessori).
- You comment on the strength of a child's red blood after an injury instead of the injury itself (like Milton Erickson).
- You tell a child to embrace the useful butterflies in her tummy rather than try to eliminate them (like Beltzer et al., 2014).
- You implore a child to stay awake with eyes open, and resist closing her eyes and getting comfortably sleepy (like Mary Poppins).

Can we keep saying that children are more hypnotizable because they already live much of their lives in a natural trance state, and then say hypnosis must only be used by those who have graduate degrees because inductions and trances are potentially dangerous? Whenever we are in a position to influence children, is it not powerful and thus potentially dangerous? Or potentially wonderful? Does the term *hypnosis* and its formal constructs make it more so? A client told me how decades ago her first grade teacher said to the class, "If you don't behave, you will go home and find your mother dead on the couch." This teacher had (in someone's opinion) adequate training and a job. I have watched a video of volunteer Little League coach Dave Belisle (who works as a salesman) talking to his Rhode Island team about connection and character after a tough loss in the 2014 Little League World Series, while modeling for them (and all who have watched the speech since) exactly what connection and character look and sound like (Kids Receive Speech to Remember, 2014).

Believe me, I fully endorse the benefits provided by training, education, and solid research. (I remember watching a story about hypnosis on a news station in Boston. My excitement turned to horror when they ended the segment by interviewing and observing a man who offered hypnosis for breast enhancement.) Knowing how to create an effective intervention that connects with the child in front of you takes knowledge and practice, whatever the context. People who know nothing about how children work shouldn't be entrusted to care for, treat, and influence them, hypnotically or not. (Of course, anyone can have a child, but that's a whole different can of worms.) My main point here is if we acknowledge that hypnotic communication happens—just as influence happens—then let's capitalize on that. My hope is that this book will normalize and model the use of hypnotic processes in the many areas where children may benefit, including parenting.

It is in this spirit that I offer you one final instruction: open your ears and eyes, and listen to and observe the examples all around you: the particularly engaging coach, the teacher who captivates a class of 4- (or 14)-year-olds, the nurse who has that "magic" way with a child in stressful situations. Listen to those around you who skillfully teach, engage, and communicate in positive, hypnotic ways—parents, therapeutic riding instructors, dog trainers, soccer and swim coaches, wizards, and dental assistants—just as I listened to Mary, my sons' wonderful preschool teacher. Then, incorporate the best of what they do into what you do. Instead of seeing hypnosis as separate, mysterious, and unique, hear it all around you—and be inspired to use it with joy and enthusiasm to help the families you meet.

Appendix A

Hypnosis Resources and Training Opportunities

The National Pediatric Hypnosis Training Institute (NPHTI) was founded in 2010 by a core faculty who have been teaching annual pediatric-specific workshops together since 1986. NPHTI offers yearly tri-level training for licensed professionals in a variety of fields, including medicine, psychology, dentistry, nursing, and physical and occupational therapy. Students actively enrolled in degree programs are also welcome. The three-day workshops are experiential and taught by many of the most renowned leaders (clinicians, teachers, authors, researchers) in this subspecialty field (for more information, go to www.nphti.net).

The American Society of Clinical Hypnosis (www.asch.net) was founded by Milton H. Erickson, MD, in 1957 and is the largest organization in the United States for licensed health care and mental health professionals who use clinical hypnosis. ASCH offers professional hypnosis training workshops, certification, and networking opportunities. It provides tri-level training four to six times a year, and approves training by other groups that meets their standards of training.

The Milton H. Erickson Foundation provides hypnosis training, advanced master classes, and conferences on a variety of psychotherapeutic and hypnosis-related topics. Founded by Dr. Jeffrey

Zeig in 1979, the foundation offers multiple learning opportunities and resources for those interested in incorporating hypnosis and strategic therapy into their practices. The website (www.erickson-foundation.org) is full of information on conferences, workshops, and other training materials.

Appendix B

Children's Books That Model Positive Frames and Skills

The ritual of sitting together and becoming absorbed in a wonderful children's book is hypnotically connecting. This list of children's books is meant to be a starting point, designed to get your own imaginations going, and I happily add to it frequently. There are thousands of wonderful books that illustrate the skills children (and the parents that read aloud to them) can use to manage challenges, develop flexibility, and revel in the unexpected moments of growing up. Offer this list to the parents and teachers you know, and have some of your favorites on hand to share with the children you encounter.

UP TO AGE 5

Brave, Brave Mouse by Michaela Morgan, illustrated by Michelle Cartlidge (Albert Whitman, 2004). A mouse learns how and when to say *yes*, and that *no* works, too, sometimes. Teaches kids: selectivity, discrimination, the good combination of risks and limits.

The Carrot Seed by Ruth Krauss, illustrated by Crockett Johnson (HarperCollins, reprint, 2004). A classic, simple, sweet tale of internal persistence in the face of grown-up doubt. Teaches kids: confidence, persistence, determination, positive expectancy.

Make It Change by David Evans and Claudette Williams (Dorling Lindersley, 1992). A science book for children with simple experiments that promote thinking and doing. Teaches kids: experimenting, change happens, taking action, cause and effect, sequencing.

Not a Box by Antoinette Portis (HarperCollins, 2007). A bunny shows that he won't be boxed in by a box. Teaches kids: imagination, versatility, thinking outside the box.

We'll All Go Exploring by Maggee Spicer and Richard Thompson, illustrated by Kim Lafave (Fitzhenry and Whiteside, 2003). The title is repeated, supporting the simple joys of exploring the world around us. Teaches kids: exploring, investigating.

Yahoo for You by Dana Meachen Rau, illustrated by Cary Pillo (Compass Point, 2006). This book offers a direct and simple message to little ones about trying new things. Teaches kids: flexibility, risk taking, exploring, taking action.

AGE 4 AND UP

Alvah and Arvilla by Mary Lyn Ray (Harcourt Children's Books, 1994). A New England couple decide it's time to see the Pacific Ocean, but have to take their farm animals with them on the journey. Teaches kids: problem solving, flexibility, determination, and the value of action.

Beetle McGrady Eats Bugs by Megan McDonald (Greenwillow, 2005). Beetle McGrady is a daring girl, who takes on the challenge of eating bugs, just to show she can. This will make picky eaters squirm, but Beetle's determination in the face of her cautious classmates is contagious. Teaches kids: persistence, experimenting, risk taking.

Begin at the Beginning: A Little Artist Learns About Life by Amy Schwartz (Katherine Tegen, 2005). An overwhelmed little girl learns how to make a big challenge manageable. Teaches kids: steps and sequencing, compartmentalization, accessing resources.

Beverly Billingsly Borrows a Book by Alexander Stadler (Harcourt Children's Books, 2003). Beverly shows how problems can get bigger in your imagination. This one shows avoidance in action. Teaches kids: action helps more than ruminating and avoidance, the pitfalls of jumping to conclusions, sometimes solutions are simple.

Beverly Billingsly Takes a Bow by Alexander Stadler (Harcourt Children's Books, 2002). Beverly hesitantly gets into the action, and discovers that good things happen when you put yourself in the game, just sometimes not how you expect. Teaches kids: flexibility, discovery, the ability to create a happy ending, the need to take action.

Fables by Arnold Lobel (HarperCollins, 1980). More tales from Mr. Lobel, with fresh and funny morals and wonderful illustrations. Teaches kids: flexibility, risk taking, the power of observation, the dangers of getting stuck.

Fortunately by Remy Charlip (Perfection Learning, 2010). What happens when you're invited to a birthday party thousands of miles away? You figure out how to get there! Teaches kids: resourcefulness, hopefulness, persistence, and the need for action.

A Friend Like Ed by Karen Wagner and Janet Pedersen (Orchard/Watts Group, 2000). Ed is a bit eccentric, and Mildred goes in search of a more "normal" friend, only to return to Ed, kookiness and all. Teaches kids: accepting differences, loyalty, flexibility, the importance and possibility of connection and friendship.

The Frog and Toad Books Collection Box Set by Arnold Lobel (HarperCollins, 2004). The classic read-aloud stories, all with a moral worthy of discussion. Wonderfully, sweetly written. Teaches kids: all sorts of great things about friendship and bravery and flexibility and kindness.

Ming Lo Moves the Mountain by Arnold Lobel (Scholastic, 1986). Ming Lo and his wife want to move the mountain away from their house, but discover that a change in perspective offers the same happy result. There's more than one way to move a mountain!

Teaches kids: flexibility, shifting points of view, creativity, problem solving.

Once Upon an Ordinary School Day by Colin McNaughton, illustrated by Satoshi Kitamura (Farrar, Straus and Giroux, 2005). A regular school day takes some unexpected turns in this wonderful, magical book. Teaches kids: imagination, possibilities, thinking outside the box, positive expectancy.

The Opposite by Tom MacRae and Elena Odriozola (Peachtree, 2006). This is a brilliant book that describes how every anxious kid should tackle the part inside that holds him or her back. I wish I wrote this book and am very glad I came across it. Teaches kids: the critical concept of confronting anxiety and fear rather than avoiding.

The Owl Who Was Afraid of the Dark by Jill Tomlinson and Paul Howard (Egmont UK, 2004). Plop the owl learns to see darkness as less scary when he experiences it from others' perspectives. (There are several other books in this series with titles like *The Hen Who Wouldn't Give Up*.) Teaches kids: flexibility, shifts in perspective, experience is malleable.

Sally Jean, the Bicycle Queen by Carl Best, illustrated by Christine Davenier (Farrar, Straus and Giroux, 2006). Sally Jean grows in and out of her beloved bicycles, while solving many conundrums along the way. Teaches kids: persistence, creativity, resourcefulness, steps and sequencing, mastery.

Snowflake Bentley by Jacqueline Briggs Martin, illustrated by Mary Azarian (Houghton Mifflin Harcourt, 2009). This book tells the story of Wilson Bentley, determined to photograph snowflakes and capture for the world their beauty and individuality. Despite little support or understanding from others, Bentley preserves and reveals to the world what we now take for granted: that no two snowflakes are alike. Teaches kids: perseverance, creativity, and courage in the face of failure.

Something Might Happen by Helen Lester, illustrated by Lynn Musinger (Houghton Mifflin Books for Children, 2003). Yep. Something might. Teaches kids: how to manage the unknown, experimentation, discovering and accessing resources.

The Summerfolk by Doris Burns (Weekly Reader Book Club Edition, 1968). A shy, isolated, grumpy boy meets a unique cadre of children, and has a good time in spite of himself. A favorite from my childhood that delights even after thousands of readings. Teaches kids: malleability of experience, flexibility, shifting perspectives, social skills, risk taking, and connection.

Time of Wonder by Robert McCloskey (Viking, 1968). Children experience (safely) a hurricane on their beloved Maine island, and then discover how the landscape changes in interesting ways. Teaches kids: adaptability, change happens, shifts in perspective, flexibility.

Wanda's Monster by Eileen Spinelli, illustrated by Nancy Hayashi (Albert Whitman, 2002). Wanda learns of a whole new way to handle a monster in the closet, and learns that worries come, but then go, too. Teaches kids: worries and fears are manageable and malleable, shifting perspectives, creativity and accessing resources.

Watching . . . by Suzy Chic and Monique Toursay (Winged Chariot, 2007). A sweet little book about patience and the joys of letting things unfold in their own time. Teaches kids: patience, planning, the opposite of impulsivity, generosity, sequencing.

References

Aamodt, S., & Wang, S. (2011). *Welcome to your child's brain: How the mind grows from conception to college.* New York: Bloomsbury USA.

Abramson, L., Metalsky, G., & Alloy, L. (1989). Hopelessness depression: A theory-based subtype of depression. *Psychological Review, 96*(2), 358–372.

Accardi, M., & Milling, L. (2009). The effectiveness of hypnosis for reducing procedure-related pain in children and adolescents: A comprehensive methodological review. *Journal of Behavioral Medicine, 32*(4), 328–339. doi:10.1007/s10865-009-9207-6

Adrienne, H. (2010). *On fertile ground: Healing infertility.* New York: Helen Adrienne.

Alfano, C. A., Zakem, A. H., Costa, N. M., Taylor, L. K., & Weems, C. F. (2009). Sleep problems and their relation to cognitive factors, anxiety, and depressive symptoms in children and adolescents. *Depression and Anxiety (1091-4269), 26*(6), 503–512. doi:10.1002/da.20443

Amstadter, A. (2008). Emotion regulation and anxiety disorders. *Journal of Anxiety Disorders, 22*(2), 211–221. doi:http://dx.doi.org/10.1016/j.janxdis.2007.02.004

Anbar, R. D. (2001a). Self-hypnosis for management of chronic dyspnea in pediatric patients. *Pediatrics, 107*(2), E21.

Anbar, R. D. (2001b). Self-hypnosis for treatment of functional abdominal pain in childhood. *Clinical Pediatrics, 40,* 447–451.

Anbar, R. D. (2002). You don't like the taste of your medication? So change the taste! *Clinical Pediatrics, 41*, 197–198.

Anbar, R. D. (2003). Self-hypnosis for anxiety associated with severe asthma: A case report. *BMC Pediatrics, 3*, 7. doi:10.1186/1471-2431-3-7

Anbar, R., & Slothower, M. (2006). Hypnosis for treatment of insomnia in school-age children: A retrospective chart review. *BMC Pediatrics, 6*(1), 23.

Bagner, D. M., Rodríguez, G. M., Blake, C. A., & Rosa-Olivares, J. (2013). Home-based preventive parenting intervention for at-risk infants and their families: An open trial. *Cognitive and Behavioral Practice, 20*(3), 334–348. doi:http://dx.doi.org/10.1016/j.cbpra.2012.08.001

Baker, E. (1983). Effects of chronic illness on cognitive development: The mind, the body, the self. In D. R. Copeland, B. Pfefferbaum, & A. Stovall (Eds.), *The mind of the child who is said to be sick* (pp. 68–81). Springfield, IL: Charles C Thomas.

Barber, T. X. (2000). A deeper understanding of hypnosis: Its secrets, its nature, its essence. *American Journal of Clinical Hypnosis, 42*(3–4), 208–272. doi:10.1080/00029157.2000.10734361

Barlow, D. H. (2001). *Anxiety and its disorders: The nature and treatment of anxiety and panic* (2nd ed.). New York: Guilford.

Barlow, D., Allen, L., & Choate, M. (2004). Toward a unified treatment for emotional disorders. *Behavior Therapy, 35*, 205–230.

Barrett, D. (2006). Hypnosis in film and television. *American Journal of Clinical Hypnosis, 49*(1), 13–30. doi:10.1080/00029157.2006.10401549

Battino, R. (2007). Expectation: Principles and practice of very brief therapy. *Contemporary Hypnosis, 24*(1), 19–29. doi:10.1002/ch.325

Baumann, R. J. (2002). Behavioral treatment of migraine in children and adolescents. *Pediatric Drugs, 4*(9), 555–561.

Baumeister, R. F., Bratslavsky, E., Finkenauer, C., & Vohs, K. D. (2001). Bad is stronger than good. *Review of General Psychology, 5*(4),

323–370. doi:10.1037/1089-2680.5.4.323

Beck, A. T. (1976). *Cognitive therapy and the emotional disorders*. New York: International Universities Press.

Beck, A., Rush, A., Shaw, B., & Emery, G. (1979). *Cognitive therapy of depression*. New York: Guilford.

Beesdo, K., Knappe, S., & Pine, D. S. (2009). Anxiety and anxiety disorders in children and adolescents: Developmental issues and implications for DSM-V. *Psychiatric Clinics of North America, 32*(3), 483–524. doi:http://dx.doi.org/10.1016/j.psc.2009.06.002

Beltzer, M. L., Nock, M. K., Peters, B. J., & Jamieson, J. P. (2014). Rethinking butterflies: The affective, physiological, and performance effects of reappraising arousal during social evaluation. *Emotion, 14*(4), 761–768. doi:10.1037/a0036326

Berberich, F. R. (2007). Pediatric suggestions: Using hypnosis in the routine examination of children. *American Journal of Clinical Hypnosis, 50*(2), 121–129. doi:10.1080/00029157.2007.10401609

Berberich, F. R. (2011). Attending to suggestion and trance in the pediatric history and physical examination: A case study. *American Journal of Clinical Hypnosis, 54*(1), 5–15. doi:10.1080/00029157.2011.566645

Biederman, J., Rosenbaum, J. F., Hirshfeld, D. R., Faraone, V., Bolduc, E., Gersten, M., et al. (1990). Psychiatric correlates of behavioral inhibition of young children of parents with and without psychiatric disorders. *Archives of General Psychiatry, 47*, 21–26.

Bishop, M. D., Mintken, P. E., Bialosky, J. E., & Cleland, J. A. (2013). Patient expectations of benefit from interventions for neck pain and resulting influence on outcomes. *Journal of Orthopaedic and Sports Physical Therapy, 43*(7), 457–465. doi:10.2519/jospt.2013.4492

Bishop, S., Dalgleish, T., & Yule, W. (2004). Memory for emotional stories in high and low depressed children. *Memory, 12*(2), 214–230. doi:10.1080/09658210244000667

Bittner, A., Egger, H. L., Erkanli, A., Costello, E. J., Foley, D. L., & Angold, A. (2007). What do childhood anxiety disorders predict? *Journal of Child Psychology and Psychiatry, 48*(12), 1174–1183.

doi:10.1111/j.1469-7610.2007.01812.x

Bogels, S. M., & Zigterman, D. (2000). Dysfunctional cognitions in children with social phobia, separation anxiety disorder, and generalized anxiety disorder. *Journal of Abnormal Child Psychology, 28*(2), 205–211.

Bransford, J., Brown, A., & Cocking, R. (2000). *How people learn: Brain, mind, experience, and school committee on developments in the science of learning.* Washington, DC: National Academy Press.

Brent, D. A., Burmaher, B., Kolko, D., Baugher, M., & Bridge, J. (2001). Subsyndromal depression in adolescents after a brief psychotherapy trial: Course and outcome. *Journal of Affective Disorders, 63,* 51–58.

Brown, A. L. (1987). Metacognition, executive control, self-regulation, and other more mysterious mechanisms. In F. E. Weinert & R. H. Kluwe (Eds.), *Metacognition, motivation, and understanding* (pp. 65–116). Hillsdale, NJ: Lawrence Erlbaum.

Brown, T. A., & Barlow, D. H. (2009). A proposal for a dimensional classification system based on the shared features of the "DSM-IV" anxiety and mood disorders: Implications for assessment and treatment. *Psychological Assessment, 21*(3), 256–271.

Burns, G. W. (2001). *101 healing stories: Using metaphors in therapy.* Hoboken, NJ: Wiley.

Burns, G. W. (2005). *101 healing stories for kids and teens: Using metaphors in therapy.* Hoboken, NJ: Wiley.

Burns, G. W. (2006). Building coping skills with metaphors. In M. Yapko (Ed.), *Hypnosis and treating depression: Applications in clinical practice* (pp. 49–69). New York: Routledge.

Burns, G. W. (Ed.). (2007). *Healing with stories: Your casebook collection for using therapeutic metaphors.* Hoboken, NJ: Wiley.

Butler, L. D., & Nolen-Hoeksema, S. (1994). Gender differences in responses to depressed mood in a college sample. *Sex Roles, 30*(5), 331.

Butler, L. D., Symons, B. K., Henderson, S. L., Shortliffe, L. D., & Spiegel, D. (2005). Hypnosis reduces distress and duration of an invasive medical procedure for children. *Pediatrics, 115*(1), e77–e85.

doi:10.1542/peds.2004-0818

Calipel, S., Lucas-Polomeni, M., Wodey, E., & Ecoffey, C. (2005). Premedication in children: Hypnosis versus midazolam. *Pediatric Anesthesia, 15*(4), 275–281. doi:10.1111/j.1460-9592.2004.01514.x

Campbell-Sills, L., & Barlow, D. H. (2007). Incorporating emotion regulation conceptualizations and treatments of anxiety and mood disorders. In J. J. Gross (Ed.), *Handbook of ER.* New York: Guilford.

Caspi, A., Moffitt, T., Newman, D., & Silva, P. (1996). Behavioral observations at 3 years predict adult psychiatric disorders. *Archives of General Psychiatry, 53*, 1033–1039.

Cassels, T. G. (2013). ADHD, sleep problems, and bed sharing: Future considerations. *American Journal of Family Therapy, 41*(1), 13–25. doi:10.1080/01926187.2012.661653

Chansky, T. (2004). *Freeing your child from anxiety.* New York: Broadway.

Chase, R. M., & Pincus, D. B. (2011). Sleep-related problems in children and adolescents with anxiety disorders. *Behavioral Sleep Medicine, 9*(4), 224–236. doi:10.1080/15402002.2011.606768

Chaves, J. E. (1997). The state of the "state" debate in hypnosis: A view from the cognitive-behavioral perspective. *International Journal of Clinical and Experimental Hypnosis, 45*(3), 251–265. doi:10.1080/00207149708416127

Chaves, J. F. (1999). Deconstructing hypnosis: A generative approach to theory and research. *Contemporary Hypnosis, 16*(3), 139–143. doi:10.1002/ch.164

Clark, D. M. (1986). A cognitive approach to panic disorder. *Behaviour Research and Therapy, 24*, 461–470.

Cohen, J. A., Mannarino, A. P., & Staron, V. R. (2006). A pilot study of modified cognitive-behavioral therapy for childhood traumatic grief (CBT-CTG). *Journal of the American Academy of Child and Adolescent Psychiatry, 45*(12), 1465–1473. doi:10.1097/01.chi.0000237705.43260.2c

References

Cohen-Salmon, D. (2010). Perioperative psychobehavioural changes in children [Repercussions psychocomportementales en perioperatoire chez l'enfant]. *Annales Francaises d'Anesthesie et de Reanimation, 29*(4), 289–300. doi:10.1016/j.annfar.2010.01.020

Cooper, L. M., & London, P. (1976). Children's hypnotic susceptibility, personality, and EEG patterns. *International Journal of Clinical and Experimental Hypnosis, 24*(2), 140–148. doi:10.1080/00207147608405604

Covino, N., & Pinnell, C. (2010). Hypnosis and medicine. In S. J. Lynn, J. W. Rhue, & I. Kirsch (Eds.), *Handbook of clinical hypnosis* (2nd ed., pp. 551–573). Washington, DC: American Psychological Association.

Creswell, C., & O'Connor, T. G. (2006). "Anxious cognitions" in children: An exploration of associations and mediators. *British Journal of Developmental Psychology, 24*(4), 761–766. doi:10.1348/026151005X70418

Crick, N. R., & Dodge, K. A. (1994). A review and reformulation of social information-processing mechanisms in children's social adjustment. *Psychological Bulletin, 115*, 74–101.

Dadds, M., Barrett, P., Rapee, R., & Ryan, S. (1996). Family process and child anxiety and aggression: An observational analysis. *Journal of Abnormal Child Psychology, 24*(6), 715.

David-Ferdon, C., & Kaslow, N. J. (2008). Evidence-based psychosocial treatments for child and adolescent depression. *Journal of Clinical Child and Adolescent Psychology, 37*(1), 62–104. doi:10.1080/15374410701817865

Davis, R. N., & Nolen-Hoeksema, S. (2000). Cognitive inflexibility among ruminators and nonruminators. *Cognitive Therapy and Research, 24*(6), 699.

de Shazer, Steve. (1988) *Clues: Investigating Solutions in Brief Therapy.* New York: Norton.

Disney, W. (Producer), & Stevenson, R. (Director). (1964). *Mary Poppins* [Motion picture]. United States: Walt Disney Productions.

Dowdney, L. (2000). Annotation: Childhood bereavement following parental death. *Journal of Child Psychology and Psychiatry and Allied Disciplines, 41*(7), 819.

Dozois, D. J., & Dobson, K. S. (Eds.). (2004). *The prevention of anxiety and depression: Theory, research, and practice.* Washington, DC: American Psychological Association.

Dozois, D. J., & Westra, H. (2004). The nature of anxiety and depression: Implications for prevention. In D. J. Dozois & K. S. Dobson (Eds.), *The prevention of anxiety and depression: Theory, research, and practice* (pp. 9–41). Washington, DC: American Psychological Association.

Drake, K., & Ginsburg, G. (2012a). Family-based cognitive-behavioral treatment of chronic pediatric headache and anxiety disorders: A case study. *Child and Youth Care Forum, 41*(6), 579–598. doi:10.1007/s10566-012-9174-x

Drake, K., & Ginsburg, G. (2012b). Family factors in the development, treatment, and prevention of childhood anxiety disorders. *Clinical Child and Family Psychology Review, 15*(2), 144–162. doi:10.1007/s10567-011-0109-0

Elkins, G., Johnson, A., & Fisher, W. (2012). Cognitive hypnotherapy for pain management. *American Journal of Clinical Hypnosis, 54*(4), 294–310. doi:10.1080/00029157.2011.654284

El-Sheikh, M., Kelly, R. J., Bagley, E. J., & Wetter, E. K. (2012). Parental depressive symptoms and children's sleep: The role of family conflict. *Journal of Child Psychology and Psychiatry, 53*(7), 806–814. doi:10.1111/j.1469-7610.2012.02530.x

Erickson, M. (1964). The confusion technique in hypnosis. *American Journal of Clinical Hypnosis, 6,* 185–207.

Erickson, M. H., & Rossi, E. L. (1979). *Hypnotherapy: An exploratory casebook.* New York: Irvington.

Erickson, M. H., Rossi, E. L., & Rossi, S. I. (1976). *Hypnotic realities: The induction of clinical hypnosis and forms of indirect suggestion.* New York: Irvington.

Erikson, E. (1959). *Identity and the life cycle.* New York: Norton.

Esbjorn, B. H., Bender, P. K., Reinholdt-Dunne, M. L., Munck, L. A., & Ollendick, T. H. (2012). The development of anxiety disorders: Considering the contributions of attachment and emotion regulation. *Clinical Child and Family Psychology Review, 15*(2), 129–143. doi:10.1007/s10567-011-0105-4

Essau, C. A. (2003). Comorbidity of anxiety disorders in adolescents. *Depression and Anxiety (1091-4269), 18*(1), 1–6.

Farrelly, B., Farrelly, P., Wessler, C., & Thomas, B. (Producers), & Farrelly, B. and Farrelly, P. (Directors). (2001). *Shallow Hal.* [Motion picture] United States: 20th Century Fox.

Feldman, J. B. (2009). Expanding hypnotic pain management to the affective dimension of pain. *American Journal of Clinical Hypnosis, 51*(3), 235–254. doi:10.1080/00029157.2009.10401674

Flett, G. L., Coulter, L., Hewitt, P. L., & Nepon, T. (2011). Perfectionism, rumination, worry, and depressive symptoms in early adolescents. *Canadian Journal of School Psychology, 26*(3), 159–176.

Fortier, M. A., Del Rosario, A. M., Martin, S. R., & Kain, Z. N. (2010). Perioperative anxiety in children. *Paediatric Anaesthesia, 20*(4), 318–322. doi:10.1111/j.1460-9592.2010.03263.x

Gandhi, B., & Oakley, D. A. (2005). Does "hypnosis" by any other name smell as sweet? The efficacy of "hypnotic" inductions depends on the label "hypnosis." *Consciousness and Cognition, 14*(2), 304–315. doi:10.1016/j.concog.2004.12.004

Gardner, G. G. (1974a). Hypnosis with children. *International Journal of Clinical and Experimental Hypnosis, 22*(1), 20–38. doi:10.1080/00207147408412981

Gardner, G. G. (1974b). Parents: Obstacles or allies in child hypnotherapy? *American Journal of Clinical Hypnosis, 17*(1), 44-49.

Gardner, G. G. (1976). Attitudes of child health professionals toward hypnosis: Implications for training. *International Journal of Clinical and Experimental Hypnosis, 24*(2), 63–73. doi:10.1080/00207147608405598

Gardner, G. G. (1981). Teaching self-hypnosis to children. *International Journal of Clinical and Experimental Hypnosis, 29*, 300–312.

Garelick, M., & Wilton, N. (1997). *Where does the butterfly go when it rains?* New York: Mondo.

Gehrman, P. R., & Harb, G. C. (2010). Treatment of nightmares in the context of posttraumatic stress disorder. *Journal of Clinical Psychology, 66*(11), 1185–1194. doi:10.1002/jclp.20730

Gfeller, J., & Gorassini, D. (2010). Enhancing hypnotizability and treatment response. In S. J. Lynn, J. W. Rhue, & I. Kirsch (Eds.), *Handbook of clinical hypnosis* (2nd ed., pp. 339–355). Washington, DC: American Psychological Association.

Ginsburg, G. S. (2009). The child anxiety prevention study: Intervention model and primary outcomes. *Journal of Consulting and Clinical Psychology, 77*(3), 580–587. doi:10.1037/a0014486

Golden, W. L. (2012). Cognitive hypnotherapy for anxiety disorders. *American Journal of Clinical Hypnosis, 54*(4), 263–274. doi:10.108 0/00029157.2011.650333

Goodman, J. E., & McGrath, P. J. (1991). The epidemiology of pain in children and adolescents: A review. *Pain, 46*(3), 247–264.

Graci, G. M., & Hardie, J. C. (2007). Evidenced-based hypnotherapy for the management of sleep disorders. *International Journal of Clinical and Experimental Hypnosis, 55*(3), 288–302. doi:10.1080/00207140701338662

Gregory, A. M., Caspi, A., Eley, T. C., Moffitt, T. E., O'Connor, T. G., & Poulton, R. (2005). Prospective longitudinal associations between persistent sleep problems in childhood and anxiety and depression disorders in adulthood. *Journal of Abnormal Child Psychology, 33*(2), 157–163. doi:10. 1007/s10802-005-1824-O

Gulewitsch, M., Müller, J., Hautzinger, M., & Schlarb, A. (2013). Brief hypnotherapeutic-behavioral intervention for functional abdominal pain and irritable bowel syndrome in childhood: A randomized controlled trial. *European Journal of Pediatrics, 172*(8), 1043–1051. doi:10.1007/s00431-013-1990-y

Haley, J. (1973). *Uncommon therapy: The psychiatric techniques of Milton Erickson, M.D.* New York: Norton.

Haley, J. (2015). *A quiz for young therapists.* Retrieved March 19 from http://www.jay-haley-on-therapy.com/HaleyQuiz.pdf

Hammond, D. C. (Ed.). (1990). *Handbook of hypnotic suggestions and metaphors.* New York: Norton.

Hanson, R. (2013). *Hardwiring happiness: The new brain science of contentment, calm, and confidence.* New York: Harmony.

Hawkins, P., & Polemikos, N. (2002). Hypnosis treatment of sleeping problems in children experiencing loss. *Contemporary Hypnosis, 19*(1), 18.

Heffner, M., Greco, L. A., & Eifert, G. H. (2003). Pretend you are a turtle: Children's responses to metaphorical versus literal relaxation instructions. *Child and Family Behavior Therapy, 25*(1), 19–33. doi:10.1300/J019v25n01_02

Heng, K., & Wirrell, E. (2006). Sleep disturbance in children with migraine. *Journal of Child Neurology, 21*(9), 761–766. doi:10.2310/7010.2006.00191

Hewitt, P. L., Caelian, C. F., Flett, G. L., Sherry, S. B., Collins, L., & Flynn, C. A. (2002). Perfectionism in children: Associations with depression, anxiety, and anger. *Personality and Individual Differences, 32*(6), 1049.

Hilgard, E. R., & Hilgard, J. R. (1975). *Hypnosis in the relief of pain.* Los Altos, CA: William Kaufmann.

Hiller, R., Lovato, N., Gradisar, M., Oliver, M., & Slater, A. (2014). Trying to fall asleep while catastrophising: What sleep-disordered adolescents think and feel. *Sleep Medicine, 15*, 96–103.

Hilt, L. M., Armstrong, J. M., & Essex, M. J. (2012). Early family context and development of adolescent ruminative style: Moderation by temperament. *Cognition and Emotion, 26*(5), 916–926. doi:10.1080/02699931.2011.621932

Hilt, L. M., & Pollak, S. D. (2013). Characterizing the ruminative process in young adolescents. *Journal of Clinical Child and Adolescent Psychology, 42*(4), 519–530. doi:10.1080/15374416.2013.764825

Hofmann, S. G., Heering, S., Sawyer, A. T., & Asnaani, A. (2009). How to handle anxiety: The effects of reappraisal, acceptance, and suppression strategies on anxious arousal. *Behaviour Research and Therapy, 47*(5), 389–394. doi:http://dx.doi.org/10.1016/j.brat.2009.02.010

Hopko, D. R., Magidson, J. F., & Lejuez, C. W. (2011). Treatment failure in behavior therapy: Focus on behavioral activation for depression. *Journal of Clinical Psychology, 67*(11), 1106–1116. doi:10.1002/jclp.20840

Hudson, J., Flannery-Schroeder, E., & Kendall, P. (2004). Primary prevention of anxiety disorders. In D. J. Dozois & K. S. Dobson (Eds.), *The prevention of anxiety and depression: Theory, research, and practice* (pp. 101–130). Washington, DC: American Psychological Association.

Hudson, J. L., & Kendall, P. C. (2002). Showing you can do it: Homework in therapy for children and adolescents with anxiety disorders. *Journal of Clinical Psychology, 58*(5), 525.

Hughes, A., & Kendall, P. (2007). Prediction of cognitive behavior treatment outcome for children with anxiety disorders: Therapeutic relationship and homework compliance. *Behavioural and Cognitive Psychotherapy, 35*(4), 487–494.

Iserson, K. V. (2014). An hypnotic suggestion: Review of hypnosis for clinical emergency care. *Journal of Emergency Medicine, 46*(4), 588–596. doi:10.1016/j.jemermed.2013.09.024

Ivarsson, T., Gillberg, C., Arvidsson, T., & Broberg, A. G. (2002). The Youth Self-Report (YSR) and the Depression Self-Rating Scale (DSRS) as measures of depression and suicidality among adolescents. *European Child and Adolescent Psychiatry, 11*(1), 31–37.

Jacobs, R. H., Silva, S. G., Reinecke, M. A., Curry, J. F., Ginsburg, G. S., Kratochvil, C. J., & March, J. S. (2009). Dysfunctional attitudes scale perfectionism: A predictor and partial mediator of acute treatment outcome among clinically depressed adolescents. *Journal of Clinical Child and Adolescent Psychology, 38*(6), 803–813. doi:10.1080/15374410903259031

Jamieson, J. P., Mendes, W. B., Blackstock, E., & Schmader, T. (2010). Turning the knots in your stomach into bows: Reappraising arousal improves performance on the GRE. *Journal of Experimental Social Psychology, 46*(1), 208–212. doi:http://dx.doi.org/10.1016/j.jesp.2009.08.015

Jensen, M. P., McArthur, K. D., Barber, J., Hanley, M. A., Engel, J. M., Romano, J. M., . . . Patterson, D. R. (2006). Satisfaction with, and the beneficial side effects of, hypnotic analgesia. *International Journal of Clinical and Experimental Hypnosis, 54*(4), 432–447. doi:10.1080/00207140600856798

Joiner, T. E., Jr. (2000). A test of the hopelessness theory of depression in youth psychiatric inpatients. *Journal of Clinical Child Psychology, 29*(2), 167–176. doi:10.1207/S15374424jccp2902_3

Joyce, H. D., & Early, T. J. (2014). The impact of school connectedness and teacher support on depressive symptoms in adolescents: A multilevel analysis. *Children and Youth Services Review, 39*, 101–107. doi:10.1016/j.childyouth.2014.02.005

Kagan, J. (2013). *The human spark: The science of human development.* New York: Basic Books.

Kagan, J., Reznick, J. S., Clarke, C., Snidman, N., & Garcia-Coll, C. (1984). Behavioral inhibition to the unfamiliar. *Child Development, 55*, 2212–2225.

Kagan, J., Reznick, J. S., & Snidman, N. (1987). The physiology and psychology of behavioral inhibition in children. *Child Development, 58*(6), 1459–1473.

Kain, Z. N., Mayes, L. C., Caldwell-Andrews, A. A., Karas, D. E., & McClain, B. C. (2006). Preoperative anxiety, postoperative pain, and behavioral recovery in young children undergoing surgery. *Pediatrics, 118*(2), 651–658. doi:118/2/651

Kaiser, P. (2014). Childhood anxiety and psychophysiological reactivity: Hypnosis to build discrimination and self-regulation skills. *American Journal of Clinical Hypnosis, 56*(4), 343–367. doi:10.10 80/00029157.2014.884487

Kane, S., & Olness, K. (Eds.). (2004). *The art of therapeutic communication: The collected works of Kay F. Thompson.* Bethel, CT: Crown House.

Kaplow, J. B., Layne, C. M., Pynoos, R. S., Cohen, J. A., & Lieberman, A. (2012). DSM-V diagnostic criteria for bereavement-related disorders in children and adolescents: Developmental considerations. *Psychiatry: Interpersonal and Biological Processes, 75*(3), 243–266. doi:10.1521/psyc.2012.75.3.243

Kaslow, N. J., Stark, K. D., Printz, B., Livingston, R., & Shung, L. T. (1992). Cognitive triad inventory for children: Development and relation to depression and anxiety. *Journal of Clinical Child Psychology, 21*(4), 339.

Katz, S., Conway, C., Hammen, C., Brennan, P., & Najman, J. (2011). Childhood social withdrawal, interpersonal impairment, and young adult depression: A mediational model. *Journal of Abnormal Child Psychology, 39*(8), 1227–1238. doi:10.1007/s10802-011-9537-z

Kazantzis, N., Deane, F. P., & Ronan, K. R. (2000). Homework assignments in cognitive and behavioral therapy: A meta-analysis. *Clinical Psychology: Science and Practice, 7*(2), 189–202. doi:10.1093/clipsy.7.2.189

Kazantzis, N., & Lampropoulos, G. K. (2002). Reflecting on homework in psychotherapy: What can we conclude from research and experience. *Journal of Clinical Psychology, 58*(5), 576.

Kessler, R. S., & Miller, S. D. (1995). The use of a future time frame in psychotherapy with and without hypnosis. *American Jour-*

nal of Clinical Hypnosis, 38(1), 39–46. doi:10.1080/00029157.1995.10
403176

Kids receive speech to remember. (2014, August 18). ESPN
Video. Retrieved from http://espn.go.com/video/clip?id=11373945

King, S., Chambers, C. T., Huguet, A., MacNevin, R. C.,
McGrath, P. J., Parker, L., & MacDonald, A. J. (2011). The epidemiology of chronic pain in children and adolescents revisited: A systematic review. Pain, 152(12), 2729–2738. doi:10.1016/j.pain.2011.07.016

Kingsbury, S. J. (1993). Brief hypnotic treatment of repetitive
nightmares. American Journal of Clinical Hypnosis, 35(3), 161–169. doi:
10.1080/00029157.1993.10403000

Kirsch, I. (1985). Response expectancy as a determinant of experience and behavior. American Psychologist, 40, 1189–1202.

Kirsch, I. (1994). Clinical hypnosis as a nondeceptive placebo:
Empirically derived techniques. American Journal of Clinical Hypnosis,
37(2), 95–106. doi:10.1080/00029157.1994.10403122

Kirsch, I. (1999). How expectancies shape experience. Washington,
DC: American Psychological Association.

Kirsch, I. (2000). The response set theory of hypnosis. American
Journal of Clinical Hypnosis, 42(3–4), 274–292. doi:10.1080/00029157.
2000.10734362

Kirsch, I. (2005a). Empirical resolution of the altered state
debate. Contemporary Hypnosis, 22(1), 18–23. doi:10.1002/ch.17

Kirsch, I. (2005b). Medication and suggestion in the treatment of
depression. Contemporary Hypnosis, 22(2), 59–66.

Kirsch, I. (2005c). Placebo psychotherapy: Synonym or oxy-
moron? Journal of Clinical Psychology, 61(7), 791–803. doi:10.1002/
jclp.20126

Kirsch, I. (2009). The emperor's new drugs: Exploding the antidepressant myth. London: Random House.

Kirsch, I., & Lynn, S. J. (1997). Hypnotic involuntariness and
the automaticity of everyday life. American Journal of Clinical Hypnosis, 40(1), 329–348. doi:10.1080/00029157.1997.10403402

Kirsch, I., Mazzoni, G., Roberts, K., Dienes, Z., Hallquist, M. N., Williams, J., & Lynn, S. J. (2008). Slipping into trance. *Contemporary Hypnosis, 25*(3), 202–209. doi:10.1002/ch.361

Klimstra, T. (2013). Adolescent personality development and identity formation. *Child Development Perspectives, 7*(2), 80–84. doi:10.1111/cdep.12017

Kohen, D. P. (1986). Applications of relaxation/mental imagery (self-hypnosis) in pediatric emergencies. *International Journal of Clinical and Experimental Hypnosis, 34*(4), 283–294. doi:10.1080/00207148608406994

Kohen, D. P. (2010). Long-term follow-up of self-hypnosis training for recurrent headaches: What the children say. *International Journal of Clinical and Experimental Hypnosis, 58*(4), 417–432. doi:10.1080/00207144.2010.499342

Kohen, D. P. (2011). Chronic daily headache: Helping adolescents help themselves with self-hypnosis. *American Journal of Clinical Hypnosis, 54*(1), 32–46. doi:10.1080/00029157.2011.566767

Kohen, D. P. (2013). Depression. In L. Sugarman & W. Wester (Eds.), *Therapeutic hypnosis with children and adolescents* (2nd ed., pp. 187–208). Bethel, CT: Crown House.

Kohen, D. P., Mahowald, M. W., & Rosen, G. M. (1992). Sleep-terror disorder in children: The role of self-hypnosis in management. *American Journal of Clinical Hypnosis, 34*(4), 233–244. doi:10.1080/00029157.1992.10402853

Kohen, D., & Murray, K. (2006). Depression in children and youth: Applications of hypnosis to help young people help themselves. In M. Yapko (Ed.), *Hypnosis and treating depression: Applications in clinical practice* (pp. 189–216). New York: Routledge.

Kohen, D. P., & Olness, K. (2011). *Hypnosis and hypnotherapy with children* (4th ed.). New York: Taylor and Francis.

Kohen, D. P., Olness, K. N., Colwell, S. O., & Heimel, A. (1984). The use of relaxation-mental imagery (self-hypnosis) in the management of 505 pediatric behavioral encounters. *Journal of Developmental and Behavioral Pediatrics, 5*(1), 21–25.

Kovacs, M. (1992). *The Children's Depression Inventory (CDI) manual*. North Tonawanda, NY: Multi-Health Systems.

Koyama, T., McHaffie, J. G., Laurienti, P. J., & Coghill, R. C. (2005). The subjective experience of pain: Where expectations become reality. *Proceedings of the National Academy of Sciences of the United States of America, 102*(36), 12950–12955. doi:0408576102

Kozyrskyj, A. L., Mai, X. M., McGrath, P., Hayglass, K. T., Becker, A. B., & Macneil, B. (2008). Continued exposure to maternal distress in early life is associated with an increased risk of childhood asthma. *American Journal of Respiratory and Critical Care Medicine, 177*(2), 142–147. doi:200703-381OC

Kramer, R. L. (1989). The treatment of childhood night terrors through the use of hypnosis—a case study: A brief communication. *International Journal of Clinical and Experimental Hypnosis, 37*(4), 283–284. doi:10.1080/00207148908414482

Kuttner, L. (1988). Favorite stories: A hypnotic pain-reduction technique for children in acute pain. *American Journal of Clinical Hypnosis, 30*(4), 289–295. doi:10.1080/00029157.1988.10402752

Kuttner, L. (2009). CBT and hypnosis: The worry-bug versus the cake. *Contemporary Hypnosis, 26*(1), 60–64.

Kuttner, L. (2012). Pediatric hypnosis: Pre-, peri-, and post-anesthesia. *Paediatric Anaesthesia, 22*(6), 573–577. doi:10.1111/j.1460-9592.2012.03860.x

Kuttner, L., & Catchpole, R. (2013). Developmental considerations: Hypnosis with children. In L. Sugarman & W. C. Wester (Eds.), *Therapeutic hypnosis with children and adolescents* (2nd ed., pp. 25–44). Bethel, CT: Crown House.

Lang, E., Hatsiopoulou, O., Koch, T., Berbaum, K., Lutgendorf, S., Kettenmann, E., et al. (2005). Can words hurt? Patient-provider interactions during invasive medical procedures. *Journal of Pain, 114*, 303–309.

Lang, E., Lutgendorf, S., Logan, H., Benotsch, E., Laser, E., &

Spiegel, D. (1999). Nonpharmacologic analgesia and anxiolysis for interventional radiological procedures. *Seminars in Interventional Radiology, 16*, 113–123.

Lankton, S. (2006). Four brief hypnotic interventions in the treatment of depression. In M. Yapko (Ed.), *Hypnosis and treating depression: Applications in clinical practice* (pp. 25–47). New York: Routledge.

Lankton, S., & Matthews, W. (2010). An Ericksonian model of clinical hypnosis. In S. J. Lynn, J. W. Rhue, & I. Kirsch (Eds.), *Handbook of clinical hypnosis* (2nd ed., pp. 209–237). Washington, DC: American Psychological Association.

Layne, C. M., Saltzman, W. R., Poppleton, L., Burlingame, G. M., Pasalic, A., Durakovic, E., . . . Pynoos, R. S. (2008). Effectiveness of a school-based group psychotherapy program for war-exposed adolescents: A randomized controlled trial. *Journal of the American Academy of Child and Adolescent Psychiatry, 47*(9), 1048–1062. doi:10.1097/CHI.0b013e31817eecae

LeBaron, S. (1983). Fantasies of children and adolescents: Implications for behavioral intervention in chronic illness. In D. R. Copeland, B. Pfefferbaum, & A. Stovall (Eds.), *The mind of the child who is said to be sick* (pp. 82–96). Springfield, IL: Charles C Thomas.

Lebowitz, M. S., Ahn, W., & Nolen-Hoeksema, S. (2013). Fixable or fate? Perceptions of the biology of depression. *Journal of Consulting and Clinical Psychology, 81*(3), 518–527. doi:10.1037/a0031730

Leitenberg, H., Yost, L., & Carroll-Wilson, M. (1986). Negative cognitive errors in children: Questionnaire development, normative data, and comparisons between children with and without self-reported symptoms of depression, low self-esteem and evaluation anxiety. *Journal of Consulting and Clinical Psychology, 54*, 528–536.

Lejuez, C. W., Hopko, D. R., Acierno, R., Daughters, S. B., & Pagoto, S. L. (2011). Ten year revision of the brief behavioral activation treatment for depression: Revised treatment manual. *Behavior Modification, 35*(2), 111–161. doi:10.1177/0145445510390929

Lejuez, C. W., Hopko, D. R., & Hopko, S. D. (2001). A brief behavioral activation treatment for depression: Treatment manual. *Behavior Modification, 25*(2), 255–286.

Levine, E. S. (1980). Indirect suggestions through personalized fairy tales for treatment of childhood insomnia. *American Journal of Clinical Hypnosis, 23*(1), 57–63. doi:10.1080/00029157.1980.10404020

Linden, J. H. (2003). Playful metaphors. *American Journal of Clinical Hypnosis, 45*(3), 245–250. doi:10.1080/00029157.2003.10403530

Linden, J. (2007). And this little piggy stayed home: Playful metaphors in treating childhood separation anxiety. In G. W. Burns (Ed.), *Healing with stories: Your casebook collection for using therapeutic metaphors* (pp. 44–54). Hoboken, NJ: Wiley.

Linden, J. H. (2011). Hypnosis and parents: Pattern interruptus. *American Journal of Clinical Hypnosis, 54*(1), 70–81. doi:10.1080/00029157.2011.566644

Liossi, C., & Hatira, P. (1999). Clinical hypnosis versus cognitive behavioral training for pain management with pediatric cancer patients undergoing bone marrow aspirations. *International Journal of Clinical and Experimental Hypnosis, 47*(2), 104–116. doi:10.1080/00207149908410025

Liossi, C., & Hatira, P. (2003). Clinical hypnosis in the alleviation of procedure-related pain in pediatric oncology patients. *International Journal of Clinical and Experimental Hypnosis, 51*(1), 4–28. doi:10.1076/iceh.51.1.4.14064

Liossi, C., White, P., & Hatira, P. (2009). A randomized clinical trial of a brief hypnosis intervention to control venepuncture-related pain of paediatric cancer patients. *Pain, 142*(3), 255–263. doi:10.1016/j.pain.2009.01.017

Lobe, T. E. (2013). Perioperative hypnosis. In L. Sugarman & W. Wester (Eds.), *Therapeutic hypnosis with children and adolescents* (2nd ed., pp. 381–402). Bethel, CT: Crown House.

London, P. (1962). Hypnosis in children: An experimental approach. *International Journal of Clinical and Experimental Hypnosis, 10*(2), 79–91. doi:10.1080/00207146208415867

Luby, J., Lenze, S., & Tillman, R. (2012). A novel early intervention for preschool depression: Findings from a pilot randomized controlled trial. *Journal of Child Psychology and Psychiatry, 53*(3), 313–322.

Lynch-Jordan, A. M., Kashikar-Zuck, S., Szabova, A., & Goldschneider, K. R. (2013). The interplay of parent and adolescent catastrophizing and its impact on adolescents' pain, functioning, and pain behavior. *Clinical Journal of Pain, 29*(8), 681–688. doi:10.1097/AJP.0b013e3182757720

Lynn, S. J. (2007). Hypnosis reconsidered. *American Journal of Clinical Hypnosis, 49*(3), 195–197. doi:10.1080/00029157.2007.10401579

Lynn, S. J., Barnes, S., Deming, A., & Accardi, M. (2010). Hypnosis, rumination, and depression: Catalyzing attention and mindfulness-based treatments. *International Journal of Clinical and Experimental Hypnosis, 58*(2), 202–221. doi:10.1080/00207140903523244

Lynn, S. J., Fassler, O., & Knox, J. (2005). Hypnosis and the altered state debate: Something more or nothing more? *Contemporary Hypnosis, 22*(1), 39–45.

Lynn, S. J., & Kirsch, I. (2006). *Essentials of clinical hypnosis: An evidence-based approach.* Washington, DC: American Psychological Association.

Lynn, S. J., Neufeld, V., & Maré, C. (1993). Direct versus indirect suggestions: A conceptual and methodological review. *International Journal of Clinical and Experimental Hypnosis, 41*(2), 124–152. doi:10.1080/00207149308414543

Lynn, S. J., Rhue, J. W., & Kirsch, I. (Eds.). (2010). *Handbook of clinical hypnosis* (2nd ed.). Washington, DC: American Psychological Association.

Lynn, S. J., & Sherman, S. J. (2000). The clinical importance of sociocognitive models of hypnosis: Response set theory and Milton Erickson's strategic interventions. *American Journal of Clinical Hypnosis, 42*(3–4), 294–315. doi:10.1080/00029157.2000.10734363

Lynn, S. J., Surya Das, L., Hallquist, M. N., & Williams, J. C. (2006). Mindfulness, acceptance, and hypnosis: Cognitive and clinical perspectives. *International Journal of Clinical and Experimental Hypnosis, 54*(2), 143–166. doi:Q63335QNV2224827

Lynn, S. J., Vanderhoff, H., Shindler, K., & Stafford, J. (2002). Defining hypnosis as a trance vs. cooperation: Hypnotic inductions, suggestibility, and performance standards. *American Journal of Clinical Hypnosis, 44*(3/4), 231–240.

Lyons, L. (2013, January/February). Taming the wild things: Helping anxious kids and their parents. *Psychotherapy Networker, 37*, 38–45.

Lyubomirsky, S., Caldwell, N. D., & Nolen-Hoeksema, S. (1998). Effects of ruminative and distracting responses to depressed mood on the retrieval of autobiographical memories. *Journal of Personality and Social Psychology, 75*, 166–177.

Lyubomirsky, S., & Nolen-Hoeksema, S. (1993). Self-perpetuating properties of dysphoric rumination. *Journal of Personality and Social Psychology, 65*, 339–349.

March, J. (2007). *Talking back to OCD: The program that helps kids and teens say "no way"—and parents say "way to go."* New York: Guilford.

Markowitz, J. C., & Weissman, M. M. (2004). Interpersonal psychotherapy: Principles and applications. *World Psychiatry, 3*(3), 136–139.

Martin, S. R., Chorney, J. M., Tan, E. T., Fortier, M. A., Blount, R. L., Wald, S. H., . . . Kain, Z. N. (2011). Changing healthcare providers' behavior during pediatric inductions with an empirically based intervention. *Anesthesiology, 115*(1), 18–27. doi:10.1097/ALN.0b013e3182207bf5

Matthews, W. J., & Langdell, S. (1989). What do clients think about the metaphors they receive? An initial inquiry. *American Jour-*

nal of Clinical Hypnosis, 31(4), 242–251. doi:10.1080/00029157.1989.1 0402779

McArdle, P. (2007). Comments on NICE guidelines for "Depression in children and young people." Child and Adolescent Mental Health, 12(2), 66–69. doi:10.1111/j.1475-3588.2006.00436.x

McCloskey, R. (1957). Time of wonder. New York: Puffin.

McKown, C., Gumbiner, L. M., Russo, N. M., & Lipton, M. (2009). Social-emotional learning skill, self-regulation, and social competence in typically developing and clinic-referred children. Journal of Clinical Child and Adolescent Psychology, 38(6), 858–871. doi:10.1080/15374410903258934

McLaughlin, K. A., & Nolen-Hoeksema, S. (2011). Rumination as a transdiagnostic factor in depression and anxiety. Behaviour Research and Therapy, 49(3), 186–193. doi:10.1016/j.brat.2010.12.006

McLeod, B. D., Wood, J. J., & Weisz, J. R. (2007). Examining the association between parenting and childhood anxiety: A meta-analysis. Clinical Psychology Review, 27(2), 155–172. doi:10.1016/j.cpr.2006.09.002

McLoone, J., Hudson, J. L., & Rapee, R. M. (2006). Treating anxiety disorders in a school setting. Education and Treatment of Children, 29(2), 219.

McNeilly, R. (2007). Night, night, sleep tight, don't let the sharks bite: "What's missing?" in metaphors. In G. W. Burns (Ed.), Healing with stories: Your casebook collection for using therapeutic metaphors (pp. 190–198). Hoboken, NJ: Wiley.

McRaney, D. (2011). You are not so smart: Why you have too many friends on Facebook, why your memory is mostly fiction, and 46 other ways you're deluding yourself. New York: Gotham.

Melhem, N. M., Porta, G., Shamseddeen, W., Walker Payne, M., & Brent, D. A. (2011). Grief in children and adolescents bereaved by sudden parental death. Archives of General Psychiatry, 68(9), 911–919. doi:10.1001/archgenpsychiatry.2011.101

Meltzer, L. J. (2010). Clinical management of behavioral insomnia of childhood: Treatment of bedtime problems and night wakings in young children. *Behavioral Sleep Medicine, 8*(3), 172–189. doi:10.10 80/15402002.2010.487464

Mendes, A. V., Loureiro, S. R., Crippa, J. A., de Meneses Gaya, C., García-Esteve, L., & Martín-Santos, R. (2012). Mothers with depression, school-age children with depression? A systematic review. *Perspectives in Psychiatric Care, 48*(3), 138–148. doi:10.1111/ j.1744-6163.2011.00318.x

Michl, L. C., McLaughlin, K. A., Shepherd, K., & Nolen-Hoeksema, S. (2013). Rumination as a mechanism linking stressful life events to symptoms of depression and anxiety: Longitudinal evidence in early adolescents and adults. *Journal of Abnormal Psychology, 122*(2), 339–352. doi:10.1037/a0031994

Milling, L. S., & Costantino, C. A. (2000). Clinical hypnosis with children: First steps toward empirical support. *International Journal of Clinical and Experimental Hypnosis, 48*(2), 113–137. doi:10.1080/00207140008410044

Mindell, J. A., & Barrett, K. M. (2002). Nightmares and anxiety in elementary-aged children: Is there a relationship? *Child: Care, Health and Development, 28*(4), 317–322. doi:10.1046/j.1365-2214.2002.00274.x

Mitchell, J. H., Newall, C., Broeren, S., & Hudson, J. L. (2013). The role of perfectionism in cognitive behaviour therapy outcomes for clinically anxious children. *Behaviour Research and Therapy, 51*(9), 547–554. doi:10.1016/j.brat.2013.05.015

Mojtabai, R., & Olfson, M. (2010). National trends in psychotropic medication polypharmacy in office-based psychiatry. *Archives of General Psychiatry, 67*(1), 26–36. doi:10.1001/archgenpsychiatry.2009.175

Montessori, M. (1966). *The secret of childhood*. New York: Ballantine.

Morgan, A. H., & Hilgard, J. R. (1978). The Stanford Hypnotic Clinical Scale for children. *American Journal of Clinical Hypnosis, 21*(2–3), 148–169. doi:10.1080/00029157.1978.10403969

Mufson, L. (2010). Interpersonal psychotherapy for depressed adolescents (IPT-A): Extending the reach from academic to community settings. *Child and Adolescent Mental Health, 15*(2), 66–72. doi:10.1111/j.1475-3588.2009.00556.x

National Advisory Mental Health Council. (2008). *Transformative neurodevelopmental research in mental illness.* Washington, DC: National Institute of Mental Health.

Ng, A., Dodd, H., Gamble, A., & Hudson, J. (2013). The relationship between parent and child dysfunctional beliefs about sleep and child sleep. *Journal of Child and Family Studies, 22*(6), 827–835. doi:10.1007/s10826-012-9637-6

Night terror. (2014). Retrieved from http://www.nlm.nih.gov/medlineplus/ency/article/000809.htm

Noble, G. S., O'Laughlin, L., & Brubaker, B. (2012). Attention deficit hyperactivity disorder and sleep disturbances: Consideration of parental influence. *Behavioral Sleep Medicine, 10*(1), 41–53. doi:10.1080/15402002.2012.636274

Nolen-Hoeksema, S. (1991). Responses to depression and their effects on the duration of depressive episodes *Journal of Abnormal Psychology, 100,* 569–582.

Nolen-Hoeksema, S. (1998). The other end of the continuum: The costs of rumination. *Psychological Inquiry, 9*(3), 216.

Nolen-Hoeksema, S., Girgus, J. S., & Seligman, M. (1992). Predictors and consequences of childhood depressive symptoms: A 5-year longitudinal study. *Journal of Abnormal Psychology, 101*(3), 405–422.

Nolen-Hoeksema, S., Wolfson, A., Mumme, D., & Guskin, K. (1995). Helplessness in children of depressed and nondepressed mothers. *Developmental Psychology, 31*(3), 377–387.

O'Brien, E. M., & Mindell, J. A. (2005). Sleep and risk-taking behavior in adolescents. *Behavioral Sleep Medicine, 3*(3), 113–133. doi:10.1207/s15402010bsm0303_1

Olness, K. (1977). In-service hypnosis education in a children's hospital. *American Journal of Clinical Hypnosis, 20*(1), 80–83. doi:10.10

80/00029157.1977.10403904

Olness, K. N., & Gardner, G. G. (1988). *Hypnosis and hypnotherapy with children* (2nd ed.). Philadelphia: Grune and Stratton.

Olness, K., & Kohen, D. P. (1996). *Hypnosis and hypnotherapy with children* (3rd ed.). New York: Guilford.

Olness, K., & Libbey, P. (1987). Unrecognized biological bases of behavioral symptoms in patients referred for hypnotherapy. *American Journal of Clinical Hypnosis, 30,* 1–8.

Owens, J. A., Rosen, C. L., & Mindell, J. A. (2003). Medication use in the treatment of pediatric insomnia: Results of a survey of community-based pediatricians. *Pediatrics, 111*(5), 628.

Owens, J. A., Rosen, C. L., Mindell, J. A., & Kirchner, H. L. (2010). Use of pharmacotherapy for insomnia in child psychiatry practice: A national survey. *Sleep Medicine, 11*(7), 692–700. doi:10.1016/j.sleep.2009.11.015

Patterson, D., Jensen, M., & Montgomery, G. (2010). Hypnosis for pain control. In S. J. Lynn, J. W. Rhue, & I. Kirsch (Eds.), *Handbook of clinical hypnosis* (2nd ed., pp. 521–549). Washington, DC: American Psychological Association.

Payton, J., Weissberg, R. P., Durlak, J. A., Dymnicki, A. B., Taylor, R. D., Schellinger, K. B., & Pachan, M. (2008). *The positive impact of social and emotional learning for kindergarten to eighth-grade students: Findings from three scientific reviews.* Chicago: Collaborative for Academic, Social, and Emotional Learning.

Pelayo, R., Chen, W., Monzon, S., & Guilleminault, C. (2004). Pediatric sleep pharmacology: You want to give my kid sleeping pills? *Pediatric Clinics of North America, 51*(1), 117–134.

Phillips, M. (2006). Hypnosis with depression, posttraumatic stress disorder, and chronic pain. In M. Yapko (Ed.), *Hypnosis and treating depression: Applications in clinical practice* (pp. 217–241). New York: Routledge.

Piacentini, J., Bennett, S., Compton, S. N., Kendall, P. C., Birmaher, B., Albano, A. M., . . . Walkup, J. (2014). 24- and 36-week outcomes for the Child/Adolescent Anxiety Multimodal Study (CAMS). *Journal of the American Academy of Child and Adolescent Psychiatry, 53*(3), 297–310. doi:10.1016/j.jaac.2013.11.010

Piaget, J. (1962). *Play, dreams and imitation in childhood.* New York: Norton.

Plotnick, A., & O'Grady, D. J. (1991). Hypnotic responsiveness in children. In W. C. Wester & D. J. O'Grady (Eds.), *Clinincal hypnosis with children* (p. 19). New York: Brunner/Mazel.

Pressman, R. M., & Imber, S. C. (2011). Relationship of children's daytime behavior problems with bedtime routines/practices: A family context and the consideration of faux-ADHD. *American Journal of Family Therapy, 39*(5), 404–418. doi:10.1080/01926187.2011.601218

Rapee, R. M., Kennedy, S., Ingram, M., Edwards, S., & Sweeney, L. (2005). Prevention and early intervention of anxiety disorders in inhibited preschool children. *Journal of Consulting and Clinical Psychology, 73*(3), 488–497.

Rapee, R. M., Litwin, E. M., & Barlow, D. H. (1990). Impact of life events on subjects with panic disorder and on comparison subjects. *American Journal of Psychiatry, 147*(5), 640–644.

Ray, M. L. (1994). *Alvah and Arvilla.* San Diego, CA: Harcourt Children's Books.

Reid, S., Salmon, K., & Lovibond, P. (2006). Cognitive biases in childhood anxiety, depression, and aggression: Are they pervasive or specific? *Cognitive Therapy and Research, 30,* 531–549.

Reznick, C. (2009). *The power of your child's imagination: How to transform stress and anxiety into joy and success.* New York: Penguin.

Riera, M. (2003). *Staying connected to your teenager: How to keep them talking to you and how to hear what they're really saying.* Cambridge, MA: Perseus.

Ritterman, M. (1983). *Using hypnosis in family therapy.* San Francisco: Jossey-Bass.

Ritz, T. (2012). Airway responsiveness to psychological processes in asthma and health. *Frontiers in Physiology, 3,* 343. doi:10.3389/

fphys.2012.00343

Roelofs, J., Rood, L., Meesters, C., Te Dorsthorst, V., Bögels, S., Alloy, L. B., & Nolen-Hoeksema, S. (2009). The influence of rumination and distraction on depressed and anxious mood: A prospective examination of the response styles theory in children and adolescents. *European Child and Adolescent Psychiatry, 18*(10), 635–642. doi:10.1007/s00787-009-0026-7

Rosen, S. (Ed.). (1982). *My voice will go with you: The teaching tales of Milton H. Erickson*. New York: Norton.

Rosenquist, S. (2010). *After the stork: The couple's guide to preventing and overcoming postpartum depression*. Oakland, CA: New Harbinger.

Rossi, E., & Rossi, K. (2008). *The new neuroscience of psychotherapy, theapeutic hypnosis and rehabilitation: A creative dialogue with our genes*. Los Osos, CA: Author.

Roth-Isigkeit, A., Thyen, U., Stoven, H., Schwarzenberger, J., & Schmucker, P. (2005). Pain among children and adolescents: Restrictions in daily living and triggering factors. *Pediatrics, 115*(2), e152–162. doi:115/2/e152

Ruggiero, K. J., Morris, T. L., Hopko, D. R., & Lejuez, C. W. (2007). Application of behavioral activation treatment for depression to an adolescent with a history of child maltreatment. *Clinical Case Studies, 6*(1), 64–78. doi:10.1177/1534650105275986

Rutten, J. M. T. M., Reitsma, J. B., Vlieger, A. M., & Benninga, M. A. (2013). Gut-directed hypnotherapy for functional abdominal pain or irritable bowel syndrome in children: A systematic review. *Archives of Disease in Childhood, 98*(4), 252–257. doi:10.1136/archdischild-2012-302906

Salazar, G., Faintuch, S., Laser, E., & Lang, E. (2010). Hypnosis during invasive medical and surgical procedures. In S. J. Lynn, J. W. Rhue, & I. Kirsch (Eds.), *Handbook of clinical hypnosis* (2nd ed., pp. 575–592). Washington, DC: American Psychological Association.

Sandberg, S., Paton, J. Y., Ahola, S., McCann, D. C., McGuinness,

D., Hillary, C. R., & Oja, H. (2000). The role of acute and chronic stress in asthma attacks in children. *Lancet, 356*(9234), 982–987. doi:S0140-6736(00)02715-X

Schmidt, N. B., Richey, J. A., Buckner, J. D., & Timpano, K. R. (2009). Attention training for generalized social anxiety disorder. *Journal of Abnormal Psychology, 118*(1), 5–14. doi:10.1037/a0013643

Schneider, S., Blatter-Meunier, J., Herren, C., Adornetto, C., In-Albon, T., & Lavallee, K. (2011). Disorder-specific cognitive-behavioral therapy for separation anxiety disorder in young children: A randomized waiting-list-controlled trial. *Psychotherapy and Psychosomatics, 80*(4), 206–215. doi:10.1159/000323444

Schubart, J. R., Camacho, F., & Leslie, D. (2014). Psychotropic medication trends among children and adolescents with autism spectrum disorder in the Medicaid program. *Autism, 18*(6), 631–637. doi:10.1177/1362361313497537

Sebastian, C., Burnett, S., & Blakemore, S. J. (2008). Development of the self-concept during adolescence. *Trends in Cognitive Sciences, 12*(11), 441–446. doi:10.1016/j.tics.2008.07.008

Seligman, M. (1989). Explanatory style: Predicting depression, achievement, and health. In M. Yapko (Ed.), *Brief therapy approaches to treating anxiety and depression* (pp. 5–32). New York: Brunner/Mazel.

Seligman, M. (1990). *Learned optimism.* New York: Alfred A. Knopf.

Seligman, M. E. P. (1995). *The optimistic child: A proven program to safeguard against depression and build lifelong resilience.* Boston: Houghton Mifflin.

Seligman, M. E. P. (2011). *Flourish: A visionary new understanding of happiness and well-being.* New York: Free Press.

Seligman, M. E. P., Nolen-Hoeksema, S., Thorton, N., & Thornton, K. M. (1990). Explanatory style as a mechanism of disappointing athletic performance. *Psychological Science, 1*(2), 143–146.

Shanahan, L., Copeland, W. E., Angold, A., Bondy, C. L., & Costello, E. J. (2014). Sleep problems predict and are predicted by generalized anxiety/depression and oppositional defiant disorder.

Journal of the American Academy of Child and Adolescent Psychiatry, 53(5), 550–558. doi:10.1016/j.jaac.2013.12.029

Silverman, W. K., Fleisig, W., Rabian, B., & Peterson, R. A. (1991). Childhood anxiety sensitivity index. *Journal of Clinical Child Psychology, 20*(2), 162.

Simola, P., Liukkonen, K., Pitkäranta, A., Pirinen, T., & Aronen, E. T. (2014). Psychosocial and somatic outcomes of sleep problems in children: A 4-year follow-up study. *Child: Care, Health and Development, 40*(1), 60–67. doi:10.1111/j.1365-2214.2012.01412.x

Sleep terrors (night terrors). (2014, August 12). Mayo Clinic. Retrieved from http://www.mayoclinic.org/diseases-conditions/night-terrors/basics/causes/con-20032552

Sliwinski, J., & Elkins, G. R. (2013). Enhancing placebo effects: Insights from social psychology. *American Journal of Clinical Hypnosis, 55*(3), 236–248. doi:10.1080/00029157.2012.740434

Smedje, H., Broman, J., & Hetta, J. (2001). Short-term prospective study of sleep disturbances in 5–8-year-old children. *Acta Paediatrica, 90*(12), 1456–1463. doi:10.1080/08035250152708897

Spinelli, E., & Hayashi, N. (2002). *Wanda's monster.* Park Ridge, IL: Albert Whitman.

Stojanovski, S. D., Rasu, R. S., Balkrishnan, R., & Nahata, M. C. (2007). Trends in medication prescribing for pediatric sleep difficulties in US outpatient settings. *Sleep, 30*(8), 1013–1017.

St-Onge, M., Mercier, P., & De Koninck, J. (2009). Imagery rehearsal therapy for frequent nightmares in children. *Behavioral Sleep Medicine, 7*(2), 81–98. doi:10.1080/15402000902762360

Sugarman, L. I. (1996). Hypnosis: Teaching children self-regulation. *Pediatrics in Review, 17*, 5–11.

Sugarman, L. (2013). Hypnosis for children and adolescents with recurrent pain. In L. Sugarman & W. Wester (Eds.), *Therapeutic hypnosis with chlldren and adolescents* (2nd ed., pp. 459-490). Bethel, CT: Crown House.

Sugarman, L. I., & Wester, W. C. (Eds.). (2013). *Therapeutic hyp-*

nosis with children and adolescents (2nd ed.). Bethel, CT: Crown House.

Swain, M. S., Henschke, N., Kamper, S. J., Gobina, I., Ottova-Jordan, V., & Maher, C. G. (2014). An international survey of pain in adolescents. *BMC Public Health, 14*, 447. doi:10.1186/1471-2458-14-447

Szigethy, E. M., Youk, A. O., Benhayon, D., Fairclough, D. L., Newara, M. C., Kirshner, M. A., . . . DeMaso, D. R. (2014). Depression subtypes in pediatric inflammatory bowel disease. *Journal of Pediatric Gastroenterology and Nutrition, 58*(5), 574–581. doi:10.1097/MPG.0000000000000262

Taboada, E. L. (1975). Night terrors in a child treated with hypnosis. *American Journal of Clinical Hypnosis, 17*(4), 270–271. doi:10.10 80/00029157.1975.10403756

Taghavi, M. R., Dalgleish, T., Moradi, A. R., Neshat-Doost, H., & Yule, W. (2003). Selective processing of negative emotional information in children and adolescents with generalized anxiety disorder. *British Journal of Clinical Psychology, 42*, 221–230.

Teasedale, J. D., Segal, Z. V., Williams, J. M., Ridgeway, V. A., Soulsby, J. M., & Lau, M. A. (2000). Prevention of relapse/recurrence in major depression by mindfulness-based cognitive therapy. *Journal of Consulting and Clinical Psychology, 68*, 615–623.

Teleska, J., & Sugarman, L. (2013). Hypnotic abilities. In L. Sugarman & W. Wester (Eds.), *Therapeutic hypnosis with children and adolescents* (2nd ed., pp. 63–88). Bethel, CT: Crown House.

Teubert, D., & Pinquart, M. (2011). A meta-analytic review on the prevention of symptoms of anxiety in children and adolescents. *Journal of Anxiety Disorders, 25*(8), 1046–1059. doi:http://dx.doi.org/10.1016/j.janxdis.2011.07.001

Thomas, C. P., Conrad, P., Casler, R., & Goodman, E. (2006). Trends in the use of psychotropic medications among adolescents, 1994 to 2001. *Psychiatric Services, 57*(1).

Thompson, A. H. (2012). Childhood depression revisited: Indicators, normative tests, and clinical course. *Journal of the Canadian Academy of Child and Adolescent Psychiatry, 21*(1), 5–8.

Thomson, L. (2003). A project to change the attitudes, beliefs and practices of health professionals concerning hypnosis. *American Journal of Clinical Hypnosis, 46*(1), 31–44. doi:10.1080/00029157.2003.10403563

Thomson, L. (2009). *Harry the hypno-potamus: Metaphorical tales for children.* Norwalk, CT: Crown House.

Thomson, L. I. (2005). *Harry the hypno-potamus: Metaphorical tales for the treatment of children.* Norwalk, CT: Crown House.

Tilton, P. (1984). The hypnotic hero: A technique for hypnosis with children. *International Journal of Clinical and Experimental Hypnosis, 32*(4), 366–375. doi:10.1080/00207148408416028

Tisher, M. (2007). The Children's Depression Scale in family therapy: Hearing the hurt. *Australian and New Zealand Journal of Family Therapy, 28*(3), 130–137.

Tomé-Pires, C., & Miró, J. (2012). Hypnosis for the management of chronic and cancer procedure-related pain in children. *International Journal of Clinical and Experimental Hypnosis, 60*(4), 432–457. doi:10.1080/00207144.2012.701092

Tomlinson, J., & Howard, P. (2005). *The owl who was afraid of the dark.* London: Egmont.

Touchette, E., Chollet, A., Galéra, C., Fombonne, E., Falissard, B., Boivin, M., & Melchior, M. (2012). Prior sleep problems predict internalising problems later in life. *Journal of Affective Disorders, 143*(1–3), 166–171. doi:10.1016/j.jad.2012.05.049

Trosper, S., Buzzella, B., Bennett, S., & Ehrenreich, J. (2009, September). Emotion regulation in youth with emotional disorders: Implications for a unified treatment. *Clinical Child and Family Psychology Review, 12*(3), 234–254.

Underwood, R. L., & Klein, N. M. (2002). Packaging as brand communication: Effects of product pictures on consumer responses to the package and brand. *Journal of Marketing Theory and Practice, 10*(4), 58–68.

Unwin, G., Egan, S., Canning, I., & Sherman, E. (Producers), &

Hooper, T. (Director). (2010). *The king's speech* [Motion picture]. UK: Weinstein.

Vandenberg, B. (2002). Hypnotic responsivity from a developmental perspective: Insights from young children. *International Journal of Clinical and Experimental Hypnosis, 50*(3), 229–247. doi:10.1080/00207140208410101

Vygotsky, L. (1997). Interaction between learning and development, from *Mind and Society* (1978). In M. Gauvain & M. Cole (Eds.), *Readings on the development of children* (2nd ed.). Cambridge, MA: W. H. Freeman.

Wagner, A. (2005). *Worried no more: Help and hope for anxious children* (2nd ed.). Apex, NC: Lighthouse.

Wagner, K. D., & Ambrosini, P. J. (2001). Childhood depression: Pharmacological therapy/treatment (pharmacotherapy of childhood depression). *Journal of Clinical Child Psychology, 30*(1), 88–97.

Wall, V. (1991). Developmental considerations in the use of hypnosis with children. In W. C. Wester & D. J. O'Grady (Eds.), *Clinical hypnosis with children* (pp. 3–18). New York: Brunner/Mazel.

Weems, C. F., Berman, S. L., Silverman, W. K., & Saavedra, L. M. (2001). Cognitive errors in youth with anxiety disorders: The linkages between negative cognitive errors and anxious symptoms. *Cognitive Therapy and Research, 25*(5), 559–575.

Weems, C. F., Costa, N. M., Watts, S. E., Taylor, L. K., & Cannon, M. F. (2007). Cognitive errors, anxiety sensitivity, and anxiety control beliefs. *Behavior Modification, 31*(2), 174–201.

Weems, C. F., Silverman, W. K., Rapee, R. M., & Pina, A. A. (2003). The role of control in childhood anxiety disorders. *Cognitive Therapy and Research, 27*(5), 557.

Weil, L. G., Fleming, S. M., Dumontheil, I., Kilford, E. J., Weil, R. S., Rees, G., . . . Blakemore, S. J. (2013). The development of metacognitive ability in adolescence. *Consciousness and Cognition, 22*(1), 264–271. doi:10.1016/j.concog.2013.01.004

Wells, A. (2008). *Metacognitive therapy for anxiety and depression.* New York: Guilford.

Wester, W. (2013). Induction and intensification techniques. In L. Sugarman & W. Wester (Eds.), *Therapeutic hypnosis with children and adolescents* (2nd ed., pp. 89–112). Bethel, CT: Crown House.

Wester, W. C., & O'Grady, D. J. (Eds.). (1991). *Clinical hypnosis with children*. New York: Brunner/Mazel.

Wiley, R. E., & Berman, S. L. (2013). Adolescent identity development and distress in a clinical sample. *Journal of Clinical Psychology, 69*(12), 1299–1304. doi:10.1002/jclp.22004

Wilson, A. C., Moss, A., Palermo, T. M., & Fales, J. L. (2014). Parent pain and catastrophizing are associated with pain, somatic symptoms, and pain-related disability among early adolescents. *Journal of Pediatric Psychology, 39*(4), 418–426. doi:10.1093/jpepsy/jst094

Wilson, E. R. H., Wisely, J. A., Wearden, A. J., Dunn, K. W., Edwards, J., & Tarrier, N. (2011). Do illness perceptions and mood predict healing time for burn wounds? A prospective, preliminary study. *Journal of Psychosomatic Research, 71*(5), 364–366. doi:10.1016/j.jpsychores.2011.05.009

Wilson, R., & Lyons, L. (2013). *Anxious kids, anxious parents: 7 ways to stop the worry cycle and raise courageous and independent children*. Deerfield Park, FL: Health Communications.

Wisdom, J. P., & Barker, E. C. (2006). Getting out of depression: Teens' self-help interventions to relieve depressive symptoms. *Child and Family Behavior Therapy, 28*(4), 1–11.

Wolf, A. (2002). *Get out of my life, but first could you drive me and Cheryl to the mall: A parent's guide to the new teenager* (rev. and updated ed.). New York: Farrar, Straus and Giroux.

Wolfson, A. R., & Carskadon, M. A. (1998). Sleep schedules and daytime functioning in adolescents. *Child Development, 69*(4), 875.

Wood, J. J., Piacentini, J. C., Southam-Gerow, M., Chu, B. C., & Sigman, M. (2006). Family cognitive behavioral therapy for child anxiety disorders. *Journal of the American Academy of Child and Adolescent Psychiatry, 45*(3), 314–321. doi:10.1097/01.chi.0000196425.88341.b0

World Health Organization. (2014, May 14). *WHO calls for stron-*

ger focus on adolescent health. Retrieved from http://www.who.int/mediacentre/news/releases/2014/focus-adolescent-health/en/

Yap, M. B., Pilkington, P. D., Ryan, S. M., & Jorm, A. F. (2014). Parental factors associated with depression and anxiety in young people: A systematic review and meta-analysis. *Journal of Affective Disorders, 156*, 8–23. doi:10.1016/j.jad.2013.11.007

Yapko, D. (2006). The utilization approach to treating depression in individuals with autism spectrum disorders. In M. Yapko (Ed.), *Hypnosis and treating depression: Applications in clinical practice* (pp. 243–267). New York: Routledge.

Yapko, M. D. (1983). A comparative analysis of direct and indirect hypnotic communication styles. *American Journal of Clinical Hypnosis, 25*(4), 270–276. doi:10.1080/00029157.1983.10404114

Yapko, M. (1988). *When living hurts: Directives for treating depression*. Levittown, PA: Brunner/Mazel.

Yapko, M. (1992). *Hypnosis and the treatment of depression: Strategies for change*. Levittown, PA: Brunner/Mazel.

Yapko, M. (2001). *Treating depression with hypnosis: Integrating cognitive-behavioral and strategic approaches*. Philadelphia: Brunner/Routledge.

Yapko, M. D. (Ed.). (2006). *Hynosis and treating depression*. New York: Routledge.

Yapko, M. D. (2009). *Depression is contagious: How the most common mood disorder is spreading around the world and how to stop it*. New York: Free Press.

Yapko, M. (2010a). Hypnosis and depression. In S. J. Lynn, J. W. Rhue, & I. Kirsch (Eds.), *Handbook of clinical hypnosis* (2nd ed., pp. 391–413). Washington, DC: American Psychological Association.

Yapko, M. D. (2010b). Hypnosis in the treatment of depression: An overdue approach for encouraging skillful mood management. *International Journal of Clinical and Experimental Hypnosis, 58*(2), 137–146. doi:10.1080/00207140903523137

Yapko, M. D. (2010c). Hypnotically catalyzing experiential learning across treatments for depression: Actions can speak louder than moods. *International Journal of Clinical and Experimental Hypnosis, 58*(2), 186–201. doi:10.1080/00207140903523228

Yapko, M. D. (2012). *Trancework: An introduction to the practice of clinical hypnosis* (4th ed.). New York: Routledge, Taylor and Francis.

Yapko, M. D. (2014). The spirit of hypnosis: Doing hypnosis versus being hypnotic. *American Journal of Clinical Hypnosis, 56*(3), 234–248. doi:10.1080/00029157.2013.815605

Zeig, J. K. (Ed.). (1980). *Teaching seminar with Milton H. Erickson, M.D.* New York: Brunner/Mazel.

Zeig, J. K. (1988). An Ericksonian phenomenological approach to therapeutic hypnosis induction and symptom utilization. In J. K. Zeig & S. Lankton (Eds.), *Developing Ericksonian therapy: State of the art* (pp. 353–375). New York: Brunner/Mazel.

Zeig, J. K. (2001). Hypnotic induction. In B. Geary & J. K. Zeig (Eds.), *The handbook of Ericksonian psychotherapy* (pp. 18–30). Phoenix, AZ: Milton H. Erickson Foundation.

Zeig, J. K. (2006). *Confluence: The selected papers of Jeffrey K. Zeig, volume 1.* Phoenix, AZ: Zeig, Tucker, and Theisen.

Zeig, J. K., & Lankton, S. (Eds.). (1988). *Developing Ericksonian therapy: State of the art.* New York: Brunner/Mazel.

Zeltzer, L., & Blackett Schlank, C. (2005). *Conquering your child's pain: A pediatrician's guide for reclaiming a normal childhood.* New York: Harper Collins.

Zeltzer, L. K., Dolgin, M. J., LeBaron, S., & LeBaron, C. (1991). A randomized, controlled study of behavioral intervention for chemotherapy distress in children with cancer. *Pediatrics, 88*(1), 34.

Index

Aamodt, S., 22
abdominal pain, 216, 224
absorption, 3, 4, 42, 86, 107
abstract thinking, adolescence and
    development of, 28
Accardi, M., 190
acceptance strategies, rumination
    and, 190
action counts frame
    chronic pain and illness, 229–32
    hypnosis and anxiety, 167–70
    hypnosis and depression, 191–95
    hypnosis and value of, 91–93
    questions to ask yourself about
        action, 94–95
    response set, 116
    What Went Well exercise, 195
action(s)
    connecting to others with,
        198–99
    feelings distinguished from, 198
    hypnosis and value of, 7
active distraction, rumination and,
    190
active framework, supporting, 69
active language, 94
acute pain, 212, 232–39
    dissociation by going to a differ-
        ent place, 235

hypoanesthesia suggestions and,
    237–39
inductions and, 234
posthypnotic suggestions and,
    238–39
seeding and, 233–34
shifting perception of sensation
    from big to small, 236–37
ADHD. *see* attention-deficit hyper-
    activity disorder (ADHD)
adolescence
    anxiety disorders in, 137
    role of hypnosis in, 28–31
adolescents
    age-appropriate stories for, 124
    anxiety in, prevalence of, 137
    better sleep schedules for,
        262–63
    history taking and, 36–37
    hypnosis and presenting compli-
        cations with, 30
    ruminating by, 189–90
    social withdrawal and depres-
        sion in, 173, 196
    see also teens
Adrienne, H., 305
affect bridge technique, 197
affective functioning, bidirection-
    ality between sleep and, 248